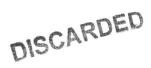
STORYTIME YOGA

Teaching Yoga to Children Through Story

by
Sydney Solis
RYT

Photographs by Michele Trapani

THE MYTHIC YOGA STUDIO
Boulder, Colorado

Copyright © 2006 Sydney Solis, The Mythic Yoga Studio
Photographs by Michele Trapani

The Mythic Yoga Studio
200 31st Street
Boulder, CO 80305

www.MythicYoga.com
www.StorytimeYoga.com

First Edition

Library of Congress Catloging-In-Publication Data

Solis, Sydney, 1966-
Storytime Yoga: Teaching Yoga to Children through Story / by Sydney Solis

ISBN 0-9777063-0-3

1. Yoga Hatha – Juvenile Literature 2. Exercise – Juvenile Literature 3. Yoga, Hatha, for children – Juvenile
Literature 4. Exercise for children – Juvenile Literature 5. Storytelling for children – Juvenile Literature
6. Storytelling technique – Juvenile Literature

To order additional copies of this book, visit www.storytimeyoga.com or call 303-456-6311

Models: Janine Hay
       Cali Machen
       Alejandro Solis
       Paloma Solis

Cover artwork by Susannah Pels

Layout by Rick Thompson

Photographed at Green Mountain Yoga Studio, Arvada, Colorado

This is an exercise program and is not intended to give specific medical advice about health. Before starting a practice, please consult your physician.

Dedicated to
my children
Frank Alejandro and Paloma Elena
Who started this all

And for their father
Frank Quesada Solis
1955-2003
May he rest in peace

ACKNOWLEDGEMENTS

I must thank the many people who have blessed my life and helped me birth this book.

First to my beautiful children, Alejandro and Paloma. My father, Albert Straub, who first introduced me to yoga, and to my sister Narada Dasi Johnson, who is still my yoga teacher and dearest friend. Love and thanks to my younger sister, Jeanie Straub, and brother, Albert Straub, because we have all been through so much together.

Thanks to my editor and saint, Eli Gottlieb, and for the many Danshube Tea House visits to help me with this book. To Alex Everitt for keeping me yang and focused; to my dearest friends, Greg Shaw, Gina Otto, Elizabeth Padilla, Bill Yesberger, Dennis Tenney, Rick Thompson, Lane Ross and Mark Casey. A big special hug to the amazing Brenda Abdilla and also to Mark Le Blanc of Small Business Success. And definitely thanks to the wonderful Michael Henry and Andrea Dupree of Lighthouse Writers. Also to Stuart Yoshida of Introspective Designs and all the friends at the Joseph Campbell Foundation Roundtable Colorado.

Thanks to Susan Merrill at Asana Studio in Golden for letting me teach my first classes there and to Juju Lucena for being my first child yoga student. I am very grateful to my yoga teacher Bhakti for her wonderful, heartfelt teachings and love throughout the years. Thanks to Mindy Arbuckle and the Green Mountain Yoga Studio, Arvada, Colorado. Thank you Frank Cochran, for removing my final obstacle.

To Bev and Tom Brayden of Jeffco Spellbinders for starting me on the journey of story. To my mentors, Laura Simms, the heart of compassionate storytelling; and Rebecca Armstrong for showing me how to dream the myth in my body, heart and soul.

Thanks to the many yoga teachers who have influenced my life over the years: Patricia Hanson, Meredith Vaughn, Cindy Lusk, John Friend and Anthony Bogart.

Special thanks to all the children with whom I have taught yoga and developed this program: The Children at the Logan School for Creative Learning, Denver, CO; the Montessori School of Golden; Free Horizon Montessori, Golden, CO; Shelton Elementary School, Golden, CO; Montessori Peaks Academy, Littleton, CO; Lakewood Head Start and the dozens of other children I've enjoyed teaching yoga to and sharing stories with.

Thanks to my dear friend since the seventh grade, Jennifer Thomas, for the music transcriptions and for keeping me young and wild.

To Martissa Spencer for teaching me the love of family. And finally, a special thanks to Susan Kaplan, for suggesting I have handouts for a teacher's conference, and I wrote this book instead.

TABLE OF CONTENTS

HEALTH and LITERACY through YOGA and STORY for CHILDREN and FAMILIES

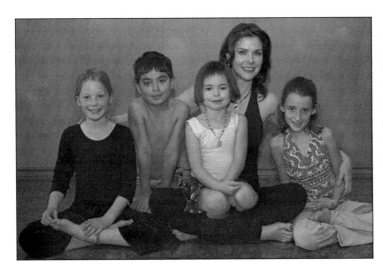

Yoga was in my life even before I knew it was called "Yoga." And stories have been a mainstay of my way of experiencing the world nearly from birth. For both these things, I'm indebted to my father. A Dutchman who grew up in Indonesia, he filled my young mind with fragrant stories of the writhing green jungle, of volcanic mountains that shook, of *babu* the nurse, the *kebong* (gardener) and living in an abandoned sultan's palace as big as God.

My mother's background was scarcely less colorful. She was a huge traveler, descended from Czech Bohemia. Her nine brothers all helped work in the St. Louis family business of painting, marbling and graining. The stories they told me connected me outwards to the world of my parents and of the past, and in the shining transparency of childhood, they allowed me to *become* those stories. So *I* was the tigers crawling underneath the house and growling. *I* was the person pouring kerosene into the cracks to kill the nesting scorpions. *I* was the person creating my own worlds from scratch.

Because he had a trunkful of books on religion and philosophy, my father also first opened my mind to the realms of abstract thought and the adventure of the spirit. In addition, his life–long physical delicacy instructed me in both the precarious nature of life, and the "radiant health" to which yoga aspires.

Later in life, enduring the traumas of which every individual existence is composed, I would be saved and enriched again and again, by yoga, which came to dwell at the center of my existence, and by the wisdon of stories. Yoga and storytelling are twin creative acts, which together tell us much about that particular condition called "being human." In addition, both are practices whose net result is an increase in compassion, strength, wisdom and focus.

Storytelling is a kind of linking — of one's self with the story, and through that story, with the wider world. In Jewish tradition, it's believed that God made humans because he loved stories. If so, he chose the right species. The human soul speaks in images, the Greeks say, and images lie at the heart of story. Personal storytelling produces the healing that is felt when one's story is witnessed and validated by another. In that telling, the energy shifts into something else. One's relationship to the material changes. It's finished, annealed in its telling.

Yoga and storytelling both also come from a point of stillness and repose. The modern world, after all, fragments and pulverizes human attention. The bombardment of media and daily life itself seems a kind of controlled violence. On top of that, science and the contemporary belief in the perfect rationality of the universe tend to flatten things, muting our sense of wonder. We need to return to that freshness of vision, which is innate in us, and is only slowly driven out.

Yoga and storytelling work hand in hand to retrieve that capacity to know awe. In addition, stories provide roadmaps, which subtly help children in making choices in life. Fairy tales, after all, involve important elements of classic psychology. Giving children these tools at an early age can do only good.

This is particularly the case now, when children are increasingly prescribed medication for ADHD and other syndromes to do with anxiety and nerves. Television is not good for kids! If reading scores are increasingly down, television, and the culture of passive entertainment of which it is a part, must shoulder a lot of the blame. The wholesale shift of reading away from old–fashioned libraries and into digital media doesn't help, either. As an inevitable result of this increasingly sedentary life, obesity for children is at record levels. On top of this, the lack of community and long hours worked by stressed parents reduces the already shrunken "personal time" between children and parents and reinforces the withdrawn habits of children needful of communication with something other than a blinking screen. This crosses all socio-economic barriers, by the way.

> *Most of all, teaching yoga and telling stories to children is fun.*

It is our special responsibility as parents to undertake the care and education of these intelligent beings coming into the world and dependent on our generosity and attention. To witness a child performing a yoga pose, with the poise, strength, self-discipline and confidence necessary can't help but arouse love and joy in a parent's heart. To see a child's imagination spin while their mind focuses on the satisfaction of telling a story is to know the magic of which we humans are capable. By focusing their energy and allowing them control over their bodies we give children the power to create their own lives and live in peace and harmony with others.

Most of all, teaching yoga and telling stories to children is fun. To be a child again and shed one's adult preoccupations is to dip one's soul in the refreshing stream of new life. In so doing, we help heal our own childhood wounds. By practicing yoga ourselves, and confronting — and overcoming — the limitations of our age and characters, we grow spiritually from the disciplined effort we put out. In the process, we suggest ourselves as precious role models for our kids. I hope that my own children can use the skills contained in this book to navigate the world and make educated choices. What greater gifts can we give our children than to plant the seeds of health and imagination through yoga and story?

The BEAUTY and HEALING of YOGA and STORIES

This book is intended for a wide spectrum of readers, and is as happy being used by yoga, gym and school teachers, librarians, childcare centers and youth groups, as it is by parents or anybody else who wants to bring the joy, health and healing of yoga and storytelling to children in their home, classroom or community.

The book employs the magic of stories, along with the ancient wisdom of yoga, to allow children to develop body awareness hand in hand with a pleasure in the use of what children, all children, have in spades: imagination. Along with this come increased self-reliance, social skills, verbal and reading aptitude, and all the wonderful things that flow from those achievements.

For those of you who are already practitioners of the art of yoga, no more explanation about this wonderful discipline is necessary. For those who are not, a few words of background. Yoga is far more than a physical exercise. It is rather a set of tools which increase one's awareness of the inter–connectedness of all living creation, while at the same time pointing the individual, body and soul, in the direction of radiant health. Yoga is a craft of awareness. When we do yoga we grow compassionate. We naturally turn toward that which is best in our natures. We experience something akin to love.

The mythologist Joseph Campbell said that the purpose of a religious symbol is to point past its image to the transcendent, before looping back into the personal. In yoga, one experiences precisely that yoked or connected feeling of the individual moving forward as part of a larger dance of time, destiny and life. This kind of religious feeling can be found even among the Founding Fathers of the United States, who nearly to a man were deists, meaning that they believed the human mind was directly capable of knowing the mind of God.

Yoga implies not only love for undifferentiated creation. It also involves love for one's self. Invariably, this process, which goes on, ebbing and flowing, over the entirety of an individual life, involves healing. All of us are wounded. All of us are imperfect. As adults, the practice of yoga, particularly when combined with storytelling, allows us to cleanse ourselves. In so doing, we are able to interrupt that reflex–projection of ourselves onto our own children, and bestow upon them a clean slate free of our unfinished emotional business. The sins of the father are visited upon the son, as the Bible says. If the energy is not recognized and transmuted, the child suffers the same fate as the parent. Yoga and storytelling combine uniquely to draw repressed emotion from where it's been stored in the mind–body weave of the human vessel. My own experience has been that yoga and story can work to heal issues which one is not able otherwise to confront and resolve. Once the memory is made conscious and the energy is removed, transformation can occur. Out of death comes life, as Christ showed. Out of stories come new meanings.

STORYTELLING

Albert Einstein said, "If you want your children to be smart, tell them stories. If you want them to be really smart, tell them more stories. If you want your children to be brilliant, tell them even more stories."

Storytelling, opening at the fifth throat chakra, acts as a primary form with which we not only make sense, but inject value into our lives. We individually conceive of our lives as stories, with beginnings, middles and ends. These stories have heroes and villains, kindly aunts and wicked stepfathers. And yet as we grow older, and become more experienced, we discover there is only really one story: the story of humankind. It is a super–story that includes all other stories: of love and hate, births, weddings, first jobs and the little things that children do.

One of the little things that children do quite early is to tell stories to themselves and their friends. No more proof is needed of story's ability to allow the human mind to make sense of itself than watching a very young child spontaneously, with no training, improvise a story. This process, when encouraged by the kind of exercises contained in this book, not only improves children's literacy, written, oral and listening skills. It also allows them to master relationships between symbols — for example sorcerers, animals and heroes — and the values for which they stand, things which, taken together, promote subtlety and complexity in a young mind. Storytelling gives children basic tools to face the challenges of growing up.

In today's frenetic world, storytelling is also about quiet time, and the peace that accrues when someone is holding a listener spellbound through telling a tale. It's about improving the home life, and the open channels of communication which are essential to the healthy grounding of a child by a parent.

YOGA

I was horrified to discover at the age of 38 that I walked entirely wrong and had scoliosis from an ankle weakness, which caused a kidney problem. It was through the awareness of my misalignment and a conscious attention to my body, emotions and thinking that within about six months of a dedicated yoga practice I was able to correct the problem. The combination of breath, attention to the body and my everyday activities combined with leg strengthening, back bends, hip openers and more, realigned my body. I paid special attention to just walking — heel to big toe, pressing off with the opposite big toe. It was frustrating at first to have to relearn something so basic as walking, but with daily practice, correct walking became the norm and is part of my life now.

If my body were to have always been in alignment with the preventative, regular practice of yoga, I would have learned to walk correctly as a child, preventing a lot of pain and expensive pills and doctors.

Additionally yoga helped my mental health. Having battled depression in my youth and much of my adulthood, the regular practice of meditation, breath and asanas combined with talk therapy helped alleviate my depression, helped me focus my mind better and gain more self-esteem.

There is no downside to doing yoga with children. At all ages and stages of life, the body naturally seeks homeostasis. Yoga addresses that natural tendency, encouraging it. Yoga also feeds the nervous system, and because it does so, tends to reduce the emotional needs which result in overeating, the literal plague of obesity currently afflicting the young of America. In addition, the discipline of yoga is very useful to a child in forming a relationship to his or her body which is not about fulfilling an external expectation. Yoga is entirely selfish, in the best sense of that word: It's "self" – ish, because through the body and spirit it nourishes the self, and does so at any age.

A side effect of a yoga practice is meditation, which is woven through this book as well. Meditation moves through the body to find the spirit, wherever it wanders, and returns it to a gentle awareness of its own boundaries and depths. Meditation allows one to tune into his or her true inner identity. Past that individual identity is that universal identity of humankind, which meditation also accesses: Love, Joy and Peace. Centered in that joy, a child's stress level drops. He or she becomes confident, fearless and ultimately peaceful in his or her surroundings. Concentration improves, with a rainbow of positive side effects in a child's life, from improved school work, relationships and creativity, to overall self–confidence and respect of others. Deep relaxation, or *shavasana*, gives children the opportunity for downtime in our speeding world, and with that downtime, cultivation of the contemplative or prayerful side. Yoga and relaxation and expressing one's self through storytelling provide a HEALTHY alternative to television after a busy day.

Never before has this kind of mental peace been as important in the formation of childhood, because the world of childhood has never before been as frenetic as it is now. Childhood is now the province of marketers, who neatly detour around parents and directly address their pitches to children themselves. The result is a steady bombardment of sound and image, soaked up by the defenseless minds of children. With this comes a real separation of mind and body, with the attention focused outward, toward the external world. The inner world — or the imagination, of love and symbols and words, numbers and concepts — is seriously shortchanged, and along with it a vibrant and independent sense of self. I believe ADHD is a result of essential psychic energy exteriorized by children who have lost or misplaced this primary relationship to their inner life. Stressed people are always tapping the sympathetic nervous system, depleting the heart and nerves. Yoga and storytelling go that place in modern childhood where calm and expanding joy are most directly needed: The inner world. Studies show that children who lack imagination are more violent because they cannot visualize alternatives to conflict. Children who have strong imaginations also have greater self–reliance — they can teach themselves rather than be forced to learn.

DIVERSITY

One can subscribe to any faith, religion or creed and still practice yoga. Yoga is not a religion, but rather a discipline that brings the individual into alignment with one's true self and purpose. The belief in divinity is a personal choice, which cannot be forced on anyone else. Forcing violates the rules of respect and privacy. But by listening to each other's mythology in a peaceful, non–judgmental and loving way the world's religions can be united in healing and understanding. The stories in this book are easily adaptable to use in a public school setting. Anything with a religious reference can be modified or omitted.

In conclusion, friends and readers, a few thoughts. Teaching children is far different an experience than teaching adults. If you already have taught children, then you know. If not, then I'll tell you that this joyous experience should be informed by a spirit of play and freedom. Patience, calm and flow are the keys. You might not accomplish what you set out to, but that's OK! Be like a fairy tale. You get what you wish for, just not in the way you expected it.

If you do not have a regular yoga practice, I urge you to start one. Find a yoga teacher or studio in your neighborhood, recreational center or gym. You might have to try many before you find one that speaks to you. Invite your friends to take yoga classes and commit to practicing together. Bring your children in and practice with them. Institute a yoga and storytelling program in your school, and have a regular family yoga and storytelling hour in your own home.

Hold storytelling circles in your home and friend's houses on a weekly or monthly basis. You can start telling stories today. Simply gather a child, children, or friend around you and say, "Let me tell you a story." They won't refuse.

The practice of yoga and storytelling has showered me with blessings in life. I wish these blessings upon you and your children.

Namaste!

ESTABLISHING A FAMILY YOGA AND STORYTELLING PRACTICE

Spending time together as a family is one of the most precious ways to create stronger emotional bonds, strengthen the community that is a family, and come together to foster love and honor between each other. Establishing a family yoga and storytelling hour can enrich these bonds.

After my children were born I would practice yoga with them alongside me. Whether they were cooing babies or 2–year–olds crawling under my downward dog, I accepted that this was the way the practice would be. You may not get a lot done, but you will enjoy being with your children in a new way, sanctified by yoga, and they will enjoy being with you. I will never forget the moment when I bowed to my 2–year–old daughter and said namaste to her. She bowed back to me and said, "Mommy stay." My heart melted, and I dove lovingly into her dark, extravagantly lashed eyes. As your children grow, so will your practice and your children's practice. My 4–year–old and 7–year–old now practice with me twice a week, and we typically practice meditation three or four times a week. The practice of storytelling has enriched their lives in countless ways, in addition to making them highly literate.

Starting a yoga and storytelling hour is simple enough. Mark out a time and day that have some calm, open space in them. A Saturday or Sunday morning or afternoon may work best.

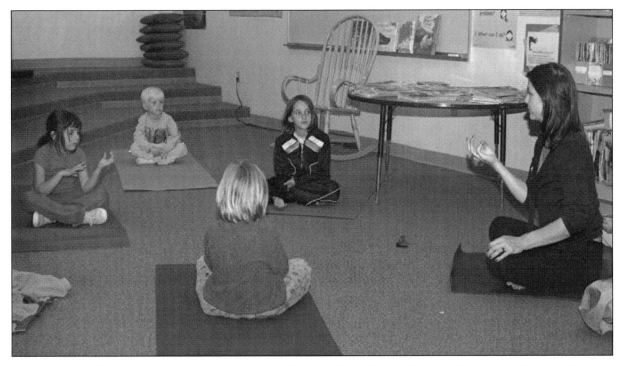

You can tell stories and practice yoga anywhere, such as the library here at Shelton Elementary School in Golden, Colorado.

Make sure, when you set the time, that it is one you know you can be consistent with. Practicing on the same day at the same time keeps the ritual alive, helps children value the practice and creates the all important force of habit.

Sanctity, ritual and ceremony are all things that children are instinctually drawn to. Create a simple family altar by gathering a few candles, special objects or family photos. This both focuses the energy of children in a special place, and may be useful to illustrate your stories. Children will learn to identify this special space with family time and yoga and storytelling time and look forward to it. After special family events, such as birthdays, family vacations, fun days or even a family death, ask children to find small objects that symbolize that experience to place on the altar. They can create an object with clay, paint, or make a craft to place on the altar. They can even draw something and fold it up and place it in a special box on the altar. Remember that the ceremonial is always important. Ask children to talk about the object, what happened, why they chose it and what it means. Share your feelings and stories, as well.

With supervision, allow children to light the candle, wave the incense stick or ring a bell. Then begin with a simple meditation. With young children, one minute of meditation is sufficient to listen to sounds, breathing, a mantra, or to remain quiet. Older children can sit for three minutes or more. Have a few warmups and then use *Storytime Yoga* or any other yoga method to begin your practice. After the story and yoga postures, you can continue with more yoga poses, or, with younger children, move into relaxation. It's important to remember that there is no goal to achieve or results to be seen but simply to BE together and strengthen our relationships to ourselves and one another.

After the yoga session, telling a few stories is fun. After a few weeks of routine, the children can be centered and calm and very receptive. Children love to hear stories, which contain within them an internal frame of reference to which young minds are drawn. A few traditional folktales can be told, or simple rhymes and finger games for younger children. Children nearly always love to hear stories of their birth or funny things they did as a child. They also love to hear stories of their parents' lives when they were young. Don't forget to tell the stories about grandparents and ancestors. These stories create a sense of belonging, identity, rootedness and continuity of the family legacy. Old family photos are great for starting stories.

When you feel the time is right, invite children to tell their own stories. Even the smallest ones can express themselves in a few words. Asking questions is a helpful way to get little ones to think. It needn't be anything fancy. A few words are fine, and older children become more expressive and can retell stories they just heard. Additionally, during the practice or storytelling children may bring up other thoughts and feelings they have been carrying, such as concerns about school, pressure, death or other issues. This is a good time to listen and be receptive and responsive to what your children have to tell you. After time has passed and there are several objects on the altar, have an altar storytelling time. In this practice, a child should choose a piece that he or she has placed there and talk about it.

Of course, visit your public library and teach your children how to read and conduct research on the Internet. Enjoy!

HOW TO FIND AND TELL STORIES

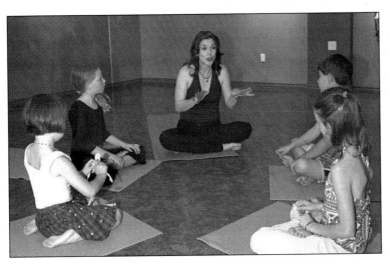

Storytelling is an art form of its own, and one gets better with practice. In my own experience, there are certain practical things one can do to make storytelling a bit easier and more effective.

As a storyteller, you are always reading, looking for new and interesting stories that resonate in your heart. Visit your library often. Librarians love to help. There are dozens of stories, folktales, myths, fairy tales and more under the 398.2 call letters in the juvenile section. Choose stories that speak to you and you really like. Look for interesting and lively characters and an involved or exciting beginning, middle and end. Encourage your children to tell stories they have heard from you. Repeat the same stories often. It's how we remember them to pass them down the ancestral line. Then introduce new ones. See the resource section at the end of this book for ideas.

Children love simple wisdom stories and longer fairy tales. The littlest of children love nursery rhymes, finger plays, puppets, songs and poetry. I always sang the Eugene Field song, "*Winken, Blinken and Nod*" to my children, as well as the classic folk song, "*Hush Little Baby*." From the time they were born I made up songs about their names and still sing those to them. I read them poetry while they were in the bathtub.

To begin with, memorize the opening line of the story. Then memorize the ending sentence. Now you have certainty in where you are starting with the story and where you are ending up. Next, start at the beginning and thread images together. What happens? Then what happens next? What is the next image that comes to your mind about what happened? Connect these images like pearls on a necklace. Or even like stepping stones across a river. Each image leads to another, moving the story along. Most of all, don't worry about memorizing the text. That will keep you stuck. Have fun and trust that you know the story. Practice the story three times in one day out loud. Lie in bed before going to sleep and rehearse the story in your mind. The story will become part of you and storytelling will become effortless and your own personality will shine through.

Have the story come alive with words that use colors, sounds, scents and other details. Speak loud and with lots of expression. Exaggerate your facial expressions for the smallest ones. Vary the pitch, tone and rhythm of your voice to make the story interesting. Move your body! Remember, it's OK to look and act silly. Kids love it! They find that when an adult is acting silly, it gives them permission to act silly and express themselves freely.

Most of all have fun. It's not important to be a performer. But what is important is having you, the caregiver, make the child feel love, security, joy and happiness. Sharing and connecting at the heart level: That's what it's all about.

TIPS ON STARTING STORYTELLING

Questions to ask:

What made you feel special today? What surprised you today?

Rehearse the day backwards. A great memory builder!

Describe a scene completely. What did your teacher wear? What did she say? What happened on the playgound today? The lunchroom?

Describe an event that happened. How did it make you feel?

Origins Questions:

Where did my name come from? What country did our relatives come from?

What kinds of foods did relatives eat growing up? What kinds of games and activities did parents do when growing up?

Pull out the family photo album. Tell a story from a photo of you as a child. Find old photos of ancestors. You can even find photos in magazines with interesting people and activities. Ask kids to make up stories from the photo, using the who, what, why, when and where model.

Stories can be built around the seasons, cycles of the moon, celebrations, special events or holidays. Ask your librarian for help in finding these stories. They are amazing!

Try creation stories for New Year's. Or make up your own creation story.

Make it a ritual to observe the new and full moon. Find stories on the sun, moon and solar system.

Take a trip around the world! Use a globe to randomly find a country. Find stories that come from that country. Tell stories about your travels to different cities or different countries and cultures.

Tell *Porquoi*, or why stories. *Why the Sky is Far Away,* an African tale by Mary Joan Gerson, is fun. Make up your own *Porquoi* story. Act it out with yoga!

Love and friendship stories are great for February. Send a wish to a loved one during yoga and meditation practice.

Thanksgiving is an excellent time to tell stories about giving, sacrifice and abundance. Winter stories abound, and for the holidays, exploring several cultures' religious faiths is a good way to develop tolerance and understanding. Select a few stories from different faiths and compare them to your own.

Don't forget poetry. Use puppets. Make silly voices with them. Sing songs. Jokes, riddles and knock–knock jokes are just as fun to tell. Put on some music and dance!

TEACHING A
STORYTIME YOGA CLASS

SAFETY

Yoga is a physical exercise. And we all know that children love to get physical, move, laugh and get wild. In teaching yoga, it's important to put safety foremost during class or in the home, all the while introducing challenging and fun positions.

Most yoga poses are simple and safe and can be performed by children. I do not teach children *pranayama*, because their nervous systems are not ready yet. For a long time I did not teach headstands, but kids love them and with proper supervision, kids can do them safely and effectively. I also teach handstands, which tend to be one of kids' favorite poses. When teaching a yoga class, and especially with handstands, things get fun and the energy level is high, so it's important to maintain control. If the energy level gets too high, accidents like getting kicked in the jaw or falling on their tummies or faces are more likely to happen.

To keep the energy level in check, it's important that the teacher maintain a calm presence. Kids can sense your energy level. Although we want to be upbeat and fun, we also want to be able to maintain order and calm. You will find a rhythm in your tellings and classes so that you will know when to bring the energy up and how to bring it down in time. Finding a nice balance is the key.

CLASS CONTROL

Before starting a new pose, such as the handstand, I gather the children around to watch me or have a proficient child demonstrate the pose first. I emphasize to children that they don't start a pose until I am finished demonstrating, and ask them to wait if they need help. I always encourage them to ask for help and that it's OK to ask for help.

Affirmation: "I can ask for help! I am worthy of help! Help me!"

I don't allow parents to stay during class. Their presence would create a conflict of authority roles, with the parent winning by default. It is also distracting for the children, who may feel self–conscious or drawn to the parent. I do hold special sessions or special workshops on occasion in which parents can watch and/or participate.

After a few classes children know the routine, feel good about participating and have confidence in their poses. They are able to quiet themselves, pay attention and follow instructions. Even among preschool children, after the first few classes, they really settle in, understand what's happening and look forward to yoga and relaxation.

Setting Rules

Children will be children. They will naturally speak, shout, wiggle, choose not to participate, etc. This should not be construed as a problem, because it's part of teaching yoga to children. Expect it. However, continual disruptions can hinder the entire class.

I set rules at the beginning of each session or class. You can even make up a "contract" and have the children sign it. I make sure the children understand the rules or contract.

I use a small ladybug puppet named Lalita the *Marequita. Marequita* means ladybug in Spanish. It's helpful to use a finger puppet to set the stage for the ritual or yoga and storytelling to begin and end. Kids love puppets. The puppet can be your alter ego and help you achieve the extra body you need to maintain order. When the rules are laid out by a second party, children respect it. I use the puppet to say hello to the children with me and teach a few Spanish words and also tell a simple poem. My favorites are nonsense poems such as Edward Lear and Spike Mulligan.

Remind children that the puppet stands for some rules. After going over the rules and having kids nod in agreement, set the puppet out near your mat. I have had children love the puppets so much, one made a yoga mat for Lalita!

When a child breaks a rule — and they will — PATIENTLY and simply say, "I'm sorry. I can't hear. Tina had her hand raised." Or, "We can't learn the new pose until you can control your body, be respectful and pay attention. Thank you."

If the child still refuses, remove the child from the classroom or have them spend time out. It is very helpful to have another teacher or adult in the room to assist.

Be aware of children with special needs. They can be the most difficult, but, of course, they are the most special. Patience and consistency will help every child feel empowered. And it will teach you a lot about yourself.

At the end of class, select children who have done well to put the puppets away. Occasionally choose a child who has shown some effort. Find some positive aspect of even the most diffiult child and recognize it in some way.

The younger or more active the child the more often he or she needs to be reminded of the rules. These are stated firmly and respectfully. The rules are:

1) No talking unless the teacher calls on the child with a raised hand. During yoga, children will want to laugh or make a comment. They may call out, at which point I tell them again to raise their hand. This is especially true of preschool children.

2) No moving until the teacher says so.

3) For children who may be excessively unruly, fidgety, talkative, etc., I make it clear that they have only two warnings. If I have to give a second warning during the first class, the child has to sit out.

   I make it clear that the child can't come back to class until they are ready to control their bodies and follow along. If the difficulty continues, I tell the child they will not be invited back to class, and I will discuss this with the parent. This can do amazing things for behavior.

4) If you are teaching very active children, start with meditation. I've noticed that the wildest children, even children with ADHD, respond to guided meditation that includes lots of imagery. Use a story or make one up. Speak in a calm and slow voice. Emphasize a focus on the body and the breath.

5) Use rewards of stickers, small objects for their altars and the honor of ringing the bell after *shavasana* as incentives for the quietest and/or most still or the most improved at being quiet and still.

EQUIPMENT

Yoga mats are very helpful, but not necessary. If possible, encourage a child to purchase a mat. They can be purchased very cheaply at department stores these days.

Having a mat allows a child to have his or her "special" place for the ritual of yoga practice. However, economics may not allow a child to purchase a mat, so I don't push it. If the floor is hard, I ask that they bring a soft blanket, and I try to have extra mats available to use. I tell them that yogis developed yoga in caves without mats, and in the poorest places, like Cuba, people use flattened cardboard boxes. An inexpensive mat, however, is a great investment. It becomes part of the child's yoga ritual.

If mats are not available, a carpeted floor works fine. I have taught in libraries, and in band rooms with carpet, and it can be a bit slippery but it will work until children are at the adult level when a mat is important to the refinement of the poses. Lower and upper elementary children are ready for mats, as they can become quite advanced.

Eye bags are also very helpful for relaxation, *shavasana*. Children may still be wiggly and an eye bag helps keep those eyes shut and the distracting light and external world out. This in turn helps them tune into their inner world. Puppets and beanie baby–type animal toys also work great. An eye bag can be easily made by sewing two rectangular strips of fabric together and filling the bag with lavender and/or buckwheat hulls. A washcloth can be used; even an old, clean sock or another article of clothing will do. Eye bags of course can be purchased. Having their own eye bags is helpful because sharing among children might cause pink eye problems. Also be sure to keep the eye bag out of the way until it's relaxation time, as children will play with them and distract the class.

A blanket is also good for children to cover up with for warmth during *shavasana*.

Drink Water!

Remind kids to bring their own water bottles, or if there is a cooler nearby, break after handstands and before the story for water.

I use a small, flexible skeleton toy named Mr. Bones to tell children to drink water and eat healthy. Mr. Bones also illustrates some very advanced yoga poses!

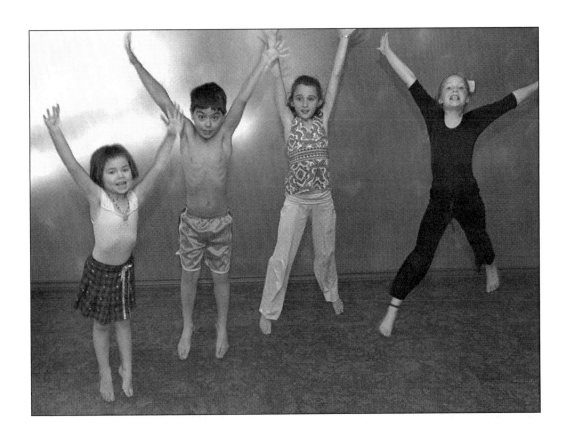

TEACHING YOGA
TO CHILDREN AGES 3 – 11

There are four age groups of children's yoga. Preschool – K (ages 3 – 6); Lower Elementary: K – 2 (ages 6 – 9); Upper Elementary: 3 – 6 (ages 9 – 11); and Mixed Ages (3 – 11).

During class, remind children to breathe and be aware of their bodies. Ask them how it feels in their toes, their hands, their arms, and their head. Remind them to keep their mind focused on the mat, body and breath.

Preschool Children: Ages 3 – 6

Preschool children are fun and sweet to teach. The goal of yoga at this age is to familiarize children with their bodies, get them forming images in their heads and get them into the routine of practicing yoga and meditation.

When teaching to preschool children it is important to teach the class in a very lively and simple manner that runs 20 to 30 minutes maximum.

Three–year–olds will not be able to hold their attention long without physical and verbal cues, and I let some children wander around or not participate as long as they are not disrupting the class, because they still take in what they hear. Three–year–olds do well when older siblings or students are present to model.

Exaggerated facial expressions and hand gestures complimented by simple sentences told with a variety of pitch and tone help keep children focused. Depending on the child, at this age kids are able to focus quite a bit.

Speak slowly and vigorously. Use body movements to illustrate the story, and encourage the children to do the same with interaction. For example, when watering a seed with a teapot, ask them, "Can you help me water the seed?" and show the movement to help children focus. Also, when telling a story or doing yoga poses, try to incorporate the three Rs: Rhyme, Rhythm and Repetition. Make up an extra song or rhyme and repeat it often. You will also need to guide them along with the story. If they can't answer "what happens next?" you simply tell them what happens. But kids can be bright at this age so give them the chance first.

When doing poses with the story, pick only a few basic ones to act out. For any physically coordinated chants, have children do the most basic movements. They are not able to coordinate their minds and bodies much yet.

We are not worried about them doing the pose exactly, or putting their complete attention into it. We are helping them put their minds into their bodies, achieve coordination and develop their imagination.

When I find a child who is distracted and not participating, I call on them and ask them to show me the pose to draw them back in. One child told me, "I don't want to do class anymore, but I do say Namaste everyday!" If a child still does not want to participate, I let them be. Usually the child will find something interesting and fun along the way and join in.

Modify and simplify meditation and concentration exercises to last only a minute or so. Always say the meditation out loud. For example, when doing the wave or counting breathing, say, "One breathe in, two breathe out," or "The wave goes in, breathe in, the wave goes out, breathe out." Allow children relaxation time for about two to five minutes, longer if they are responding well. I've had children fall asleep in my classes, which is great!

After a few classes, kids pick up the class routine and make improvements in concentration, attention and relaxation. Ask children how they feel after an exercise or meditation. It allows them to practice verbal expression and awareness of their emotions and feelings.

During class you may not notice the effect of yoga and story, but parents report that children repeat things back to them at home, whether it's a story, song, pose or meditation.

Lower Elementary: ages 6 – 9

Children at this age have better body coordination and attention spans and are able to grasp longer stories, exercises and meditations. Classes can run from 30, 45 or even 75 minutes with room for games and races. And kids love races.

Allow time for kids to joke, laugh and talk because that's the way they are at this age. The goal is to have fun and fit in what you can. Regardless, make sure a relaxation and meditation is part of class.

Children this age love stories, songs and games, which serve an important function in developing imagination. At this age they are able to recall a story, and can also make up stories using the poses.

Introducing specific poses, correcting alignment and aiding in the execution of the pose is now possible and should be incorporated during class. I am not rigid about structure or exact poses. I demonstrate the proper alignment, and make suggestions, but I don't make it a constant focus so as not to discourage the child.

Children can also lead the sun salutation, chant or recall a story. I've had children as young as four do this.

Upper Elementary: ages 8 – 11

In this age group, the class can move a little bit slower and focus more on meditation, inner awareness and also the poses themselves. More time can be spent asking children how they feel and having story discussion. Class time can run from 45 to 90 minutes, with the end of class used for more story–making discussion after *shavasana*.

At first glance, it seems that at this age children are more serious and savvy. Don't let that fool you! They still love to have fun and sing songs, hear stories and do chants. I still make silly faces, teach fun games and tell stories while incorporating a serious yoga practice. At this age, using storytelling for theme setting is possible. Ask the children to contemplate the moral or metaphor and use affirmations and reminders during practice. Suggest that they really feel inside the body, be comfortable with their bodies and internalize the process.

Children can verbalize their feelings and images better after a visualization or relaxation. They may bring up joyful things, or difficult things, such as death or a problem at school, and they have very rich imaginations.

Children are very good at recalling and retelling stories, and probably have an, "Oh, I know that story. Here's another version!" They are also excellent at creating warmups and their own stories with yoga poses.

Poses in a story can be added with an extra downward dog, forward bend, cobra, or anything you feel to get a more flowing, *vinyasa*, practice. Correct alignment is emphasized.

Children can lead the sun salutation, chant or warmup. They can also make up their own story or fairy tale through *shavasana*, add poses to the story and teach the class their story.

Be sure to add advanced poses to these children's practice as you see appropriate. Children this age can amaze you, and keep encouraging them to do the yoga so that they can do these poses and be healthy as adults.

Mixed Ages: 3 – 11

It is easiest to have classes separated by age groups, but mixed ages from 3–11 does work, especially if older siblings are involved. But you may have to separate them if behavior warrants. The three–year–olds may wander around or make the yoga mat into a blanket, but it's OK as long as they are not too disruptive. Being in the environment helps them a great deal, and I find that they do eventually participate.

Kids four and up will follow older children's modeling and the older children enjoy the role of being looked up to and helping the teacher. The older children can assist the younger children and also teach part of the class.

Classes can be extended and modified according to the development and ability of the children.

Including All Children

Boys, especially older ones, may be reluctant to participate at first, but they have always joined in once they saw how much fun the class was.

For shy kids, let them be and let them watch. Eventually they will feel safe enough to join in.

For children with ADHD start with a meditation and emphasize the body and breath during class. Remind them to bring their minds and energy down into their body. Extra time for relaxation is important, and so is covering their eyes. Walking meditation is helpful as well.

Using Affirmations

We are what we think. Negative thinking can be programmed into us through family and friends, and we reinforce that thinking when we believe them. Negative thinking causes self–criticism and self–loathing, which in turn are projected out into the world, creating bullying, authoritarianism, and violence. Negative thinking also may be related to specific diseases in the body. However, do not deny or put down any negative aspects of yourself or the children. Urge children to recognize them and set out to improve them. Emphasize that they are part of you, in this world of duality. We embrace them, but our hearts speak to a higher idea. Rejecting any part of ourselves only creates a psychological split. It's best to keep conscious of the repressed sides of ourselves through ritual and community support. We can start this by stressing to children that our emotions, the difficulties of life, are nothing to be denied or ignored. They are legitimate emotions that make up our human experience. We can recognize them and express them, and receive a return that is conscious and healthy in relation to one's environment.

The more we can use positive affirmations to counter negative thinking, the healthier we will be as children and adults. Mantras are used in yoga for engaging positive thought. They are similar to prayers. They protect the mind from negative thinking and also develop concentration. Replace every negative thought with a positive one. See how quickly your feelings about yourself and your life situation change.

During class with children, use positive affirmations freely. For example, when in mountain pose, *tadasana*, call out and have children repeat, "I am strong! I am steady! I am powerful! I believe in myself!" When in a hero pose call out, "I can do it! I love myself!" Even in concentration and relaxation exercises, children can say to themselves, "I am calm. I am peace. I am relaxed. I am OK." The more positive we can be the better.

You can help children develop their own affirmations to use through the week. Ask them about something that they don't like about themselves or want to improve or even a desire that they have. Turn it into an affirmation. For example, if a child doesn't think they are smart enough or are afraid to take a test, teach them to say, "I am smart. I am confident. I believe in myself. I can take the test easily and I will pass."

Some Affirmations:

> I trust myself.
> I love myself.
> I am powerful and strong.
> I am calm.
> I am peaceful.
> I am intelligent.
> I am worthy.
> I am wise.
> My opinions matter.
> I am kind, courteous, and gracious.
> Abundance is mine.

Principals of Yoga Alignment – based on Anusara yoga

1) Open to grace. Breathing in and filling up with the beauty of ourselves, the gift and promise of now and our divine potential. It is also opening up to something greater than ourselves, beyond form and limitation.

   In standing position, mountain pose, *tadasana*, the feet are fist–width apart, with the second toe lined up with the middle of the ankle. Feet, ankles and legs are strong, hugging the muscles to the bones, kneecaps lifted, drawing energy from the feet to the core of the pelvic area and back again to the feet and earth.

2) Muscular energy is achieved by drawing the muscles in toward each other.

3) Inner and 4) Outer Spiral is achieved by moving the inner thighs back, keeping them back, then tucking the tailbone.

5) Organic energy is achieved by extending out through the muscles and the bones, shining the great, beautiful and powerful energy that we are out into the world.

   Shoulders should be on the back. Have children shrug their shoulders by their ears, then take the shoulders back. There should not be a "banana back" with the lower back way in. The back should be full. The tailbone should be tucked and the kidney area should be full.

   In bent–knee poses, such as lunges, knees should be 90 degrees over the ankles.

   When in table position, children's fingers should be spread wide, like the rays of the sun, and wrist joints straight across.

CLASS CURRICULUM

30–minute to 45–minute class for ages 3 – 11

1) Introductory games/Checking in. Class story/Theme introduction
2) Namaste song/Breathing song
3) Centering meditation/Safe place
4) Warmups
5) Sun Salutations
6) Handstands
7) Story
8) Story retelling through yoga postures
9) Choose among games, races activities, dancing if time allows
10) Meditation — basic meditation, concentration exercises as well as guided imagery/story
11) Relaxation/*shavasana*
12) Children retell story
13) Favorite pose to do at home
14) Namaste/Closure

Encourage children to do yoga at home, at least one pose with family, and to tell the story to family members.

45–minute to 75–minute class for ages K – 6

1) Introductory games/Checking in
2) Namaste song/Breathing song
3) Centering meditation/Safe place
4) Warmups
   a) Have children make up their own warmups and teach the class.
5) Sun Salutations
6) Handstands
7) Story
8) Story retelling through yoga postures
   a) Give extra attention to correction of postures.
   b) Favorite yoga pose.
   c) Introduce one specific pose and its correct use and benefits.
   d) Add additional poses, variations to poses. For example, add a twist and a warrior pose to sun salutations.
   e) Children make up story as they go along with yoga poses.
9) Choose among games, races, activities, dancing
10) Meditation – basic meditation, concentration exercises as well as guided imagery

11) Relaxation/*shavasana*
    a) After relaxation period, introduce guided imagery — create fairy tales.
    b) Have children discuss how they felt, what images, associations, etc. Try and
       have them make a story and continue adding onto imaginative elements.
12) Children retell story or tell their own created story
13) Namaste/Closure

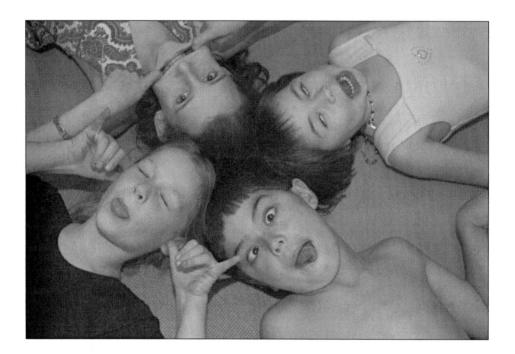

BEGINNINGS and INTRODUCTIONS

Arrange the class in a circle. For the very first class introduce yourself, then ask children to introduce themselves, give their name, age, name of teacher, favorite flavor of ice cream, favorite color or any other little fun fact they want to tell the class. Find out if they have any injuries or illness. Ask them to dedicate their practice to someone they love.

Sometimes kids will talk about difficult feelings or something that is going on in their life at the moment, such as a family member's illness or death. The beginning of class is a good time to talk about those feelings, especially if it may relate to the class story.

Introductory Exercises

Ritual

For the youngest children, use a small finger puppet to signify that yoga class will begin. Let the children know that while the puppet is out we pay attention, don't interrupt and don't bother our neighbor. Then set the puppet down at the front of your mat or somewhere the children won't disturb it.

For older children, you could use a small doll, puppet or other object, or ring a bell. Ring the bell at the end of class, and/or put away the object to signify the end of the ritual. I use a small ladybug puppet, called Lalita the *Marequita*. Kids of all ages love her, as she teaches the kids a few words in Spanish and also usually tells a poem. Children have learned to love poetry from Lalita!

Namaste Song – see appendix for words and music

Explain to children that namaste means that I bow to the goodness, light and divinity that is inside of you and that you in turn are bowing to your neighbor and recognizing the goodness, light and divinity in him or her. Also, I tell them that it is about respecting the other.

Hands are in prayer position, *anjali mudra*, in front of heart.

Children bow to each other and themselves.

Monkey on a Leash

Explain that the mind is like a little monkey jumping around from tree to tree. Have them put a leash on their monkey by reaching up into the sky with their arms, breathing in, and then breathing out as they bring the monkey down to the body, down to the breath, using the namaste, hands into heart position.

Kite

The mind can be like a kite. The wind takes it far, far away from the body. Have kids reel in their kites, reel in their minds, close to their body. Have children reach up into the sky with their arms, breathing in, and then breathing out as they bring the kite down to the body, down to the breath, hands into prayer position, *anjali mudra*.

Scattered Energy

Tell children that their energy and thoughts can be scattered out high above them. Have them stand on their tiptoes and reach up high with their hands to gather up all the scattered energy above them. Have them breathe in deep, then bring all that energy down into their bodies and heart to the prayer position, *anjali mudra*.

Tell them that they have the power to create anything they want in their life when they are focused. It's like pruning a tree, so that we get the biggest fruit from the fewest branches. This is especially good for ADHD kids.

Happy

Notice children's sitting posture. Typically their shoulders are slumped, closing off their heart.

Say, "Do I look happy?" and exaggerate your shoulders rounded and closing off your heart.

Kids will say, "NO!"

Then, sitting up tall and straight, shoulders on the back, say,

"Now do I look happy?"

Children will say, "YES!"

Have them all sit up straight, shoulders on the back, heart open.

I am happy!

I like myself!

My heart is open!

I am brave!

In seated and standing positions, periodically remind children if they are slumped, "Are you happy?" And they will fix their posture.

Om Chanting

Tell children that Om is the sound of the universe. It is the sound of creation, preservation and destruction.

Begin by chanting three oms (a – u – m).

Ocean of Oms

Each begins chanting Om at their own pace, but at the end of each Om, each student continues the Om chanting, regardless if others have finished or started again before them. The goal is to have a continuous sound of Om for a minute.

Negativity Release

Have children sit in a cross–legged position. Have them close their eyes and extend both arms out to the sides, fingertips touching the floor. Ask them to think of and visualize everything that they don't like, any negative thoughts, any problems that they brought with them to class or home today. Have them imagine those difficult and negative thoughts as big black balls. Each time they inhale, have them visualize that they are releasing the black balls. On the exhalation, the black balls roll down their arms and disappear. Repeat breathing five or six times. Emphasize the visualization of their troubles rolling off them and disappearing.

CENTERINGS – GOING WITHIN

Take a few minutes after the happy sitting for children to quiet themselves, close their eyes and place a hand on the heart. Let them imagine a special place that feels safe. It may be their house, under a tree, in their mother's arms, under the bed. Have them picture it vividly in their minds. What does it smell like? What objects are there? Can you touch them? Have the children feel the safety and sense of being special. Tell them that this safe space is always there, waiting for them in their heart. All they have to do is breathe and know that it is there. Use this safe space exercise during relaxation so children don't fear letting go or visualizing. Ask them to share the story of what they saw and felt during this exercise.

PRESCHOOL and UP CENTERINGS

Ask children to quiet themselves, close their eyes, and connect to their breath. Call out for them, breathing in — breathing out. Breathing in — breathing out.

Heart Warming

In seated position, shoulders back and the heart open. The neck is lengthened. Rub hands together. Have children feel the heat and energy in their hands. Take right hand and rub heart area clockwise. Rub hands together again. Take left hand and rub heart counter–clockwise. Ask how they feel. Ask them to try and feel their heartbeat.

Variation: Have children place opposite hand on their tummies and rub.

Flower

Imagine a little flower. What kind of a flower is it? See the little flower opening up, petal by petal. Smell the beautiful flower.

Butterfly

See a little butterfly, fluttering from flower to flower. Finally the butterfly finds a nice flower and rests. It is quiet, beautiful and happy. Imagine the butterfly completely still. Smile at the butterfly. Smile at yourself.

Big Sky

In your mind's eye look up at the sky. See it beautiful and bright blue without any clouds. It's so wide and open. Now see a little black dot up there. Watch that little dot with your mind's eye.

Little Leaves

See a beautiful tree. What kind of tree is it? See the leaves shimmering in the wind. They are beautiful and alive, just like you are. Now see the little tree stop moving. All the little leaves are still. Can you make every leaf still?

Special Person

See somebody you love in your mind's eye. Breathe in and feel the love they give you. Breathe out and send them love. Feel the love. Know that you are loved.

White Cloud

Every time you breathe in, see a little white cloud come in your nostrils. Then on the exhale, the white cloud flows out your nostrils. Repeat. In and out goes the white cloud.

Ball of Energy

Hold both hands straight out in front of you, elbows bent, palms facing. Imagine that there is a ball of energy between your hands. Have your hands about a foot apart and hold that ball of energy as if you could really feel it. Rotate the hands around that ball of energy so that one hand comes on top and another comes on the bottom of the ball. Rotate the hands around again toward the opposite direction.

Variation: Sticky ball. Pretend that the ball of energy is sticky gum. Pull your hands away from each other and feel the sticky gum on your hands, as it pulls the hands together, and then pull the hands apart again. The sticky gum pulls the hands together, and you pull them apart again.

K–6 CENTERINGS

Peaceful Garden

See a beautiful garden in your mind's eye. In that garden is a lovely chair just for you. Lovely flowers surround it. What kinds of flowers are there? Animals come around you. What kinds of animals are there? Beautiful sunlight shines on them and you. You are warm and happy. Everything is so peaceful and calm. Everything is all right.

Pond

A beautiful pond is nearby. Look at the pond. See a little bug jump in and ripple the pond. Watch as each ripple disappears and the pond becomes completely still. Watch the still pond, unmoving, peaceful and calm.

Spider Web

See a nice little spider at the center of your heart. Then the little spider sends out little threads as it makes a web. The threads connect to other threads and the web gets bigger and bigger and bigger, connecting around and around in a circle. Know that everything came from that center where the spider started. Breathe in and feel that center in your heart. Feel its peace. Breathe out and create that spider web some more, sending out your creation. Color and decorate the web. See that it is connected to everything, and that everything connects back to its center, your heart.

THOUGHT–WATCHING EXERCISES

Gardening Our Thoughts

Have children be a thought gardener in their lives by watching their own thinking. Every time they may say, "I'm stupid, ugly, worried, etc." during the day, have them note how it feels. Tell them to switch their thinking to "I am beautiful, smart, confident, etc." Encourage them to always be the gardener watching their thoughts.

Gardening Meditation

When a negative thought comes up, teach children to stop the thinking and, instead, have them imagine and even physically toss some seeds out of their hands in front of them into their garden. These seeds, tell them, are happy-thought seeds that we are planting and allowing to take root. Plant these seeds: I am happy. I am organized. I am calm, smart, focused, etc.

Teach them to replace negative thinking instantly with the happy–seed thinking. Teach them to see the seeds growing into everything they ever want and can imagine. Have them see all their dreams of happiness coming true.

MANTRAS

Mantras are helpful to focus the mind. They also protect the mind from negativity. Do a minute or two of mantra according to your beliefs. For instance, you can chant three Oms, or you can have children continuously chant Om at their own pace for 30 seconds to a minute.

OM – tell children that Om is the sound of the universe.
OM, SHANTI – Peace
OM, NAMA SHIVAYA – Salutations to Lord Shiva, who creates all of the universe.
OM, MANI PADME HUM – I am the jewel in the lotus.
SO HUM – The sound of the breath. Breathe in for So, out for Hum. Helps calm the mind.
Peace, love, peace, love
Mary, Jesus, Ave Maria
Allah Akbara – God is great.
Shalom – Peace

CHAKRA CHANT with BIJA MANTRAS

Make up a catchy tune to go with this chant. Say the first part, then have children repeat it back to you. Continue with the second and third parts, again with children repeating it back to you.

The first chakra is earth. Its color is red. The first chakra is at the base of the spine. Its sound is LAM.

The second chakra is water. Its color is orange. The second chakra is in the hips. Its sound is VAM.

The third chakra is fire. Its color is yellow. The third chakra is in the naval plexus. Its sound is RAM.

The fourth chakra is air. Its color is green. The fourth chakra is in the heart. Its sound is YAM.

The fifth chakra is ether. Its color is blue. The fifth chakra is in the throat. Its sound is HAM.

The sixth chakra is space. Its color is indigo. The sixth chakra is between the eyebrows. Its sound is OM.

The seventh chakra is beyond everything. Its color is violet. The seventh chakra is at the crown of the head. Its sound is ……… (silence). Have children hear the beat in silence.

INTRO GAMES

Face Game

In a circle the first child makes a funny face to the child next to him or her. The child receiving the face has to mimic the face back to the first child. The receiving child then turns to the child next to him or her and makes up a new funny face, continuing around the circle.

Digging Game

In a circle the first child does a non–verbal action such as digging. The child to the right of him has to guess what he is doing and name it. That child then creates his own action for the next child to guess, and the cycle continues around the circle.

Variation: Teacher creates non–verbal action, such as digging. Child to right joins in action. After that child has begun digging and continues digging, next child does the action, and so on until it flows around the whole circle back to the teacher. The teacher then changes the action, such as climbing, and each child follows the new action as it comes around the circle and back to the teacher.

Imaginary Ball Game

Have a child throw an imaginary ball to another child. Encourage them to smack it, flick it, bounce it, slowly roll it, anyway they want with any part of their body. Receiving it, the child can catch it any way she wants to. It helps to name the child who will receive the ball.

Seed Watering

Each child picks someone and turns to him. Taking turns, each child says something nice about the other: Something he does well, the way he looks, something nice about his personality, etc.

BREATH AWARENESS

Breathing Chant – see appendix for music

Have children put hands on their ribs or on their heart and stomach. At the end of each phrase, either inhale or exhale through the nose.

Remind children that if they are breathing, they are alive! Periodically ask them, "If you're breathing, what are you?"

They will learn to answer, "We're alive! It's great to be alive! It's great to be me!"

I am breathing in – breathe in
I am breathing out – breathe out
I am happy – breathe in
Oh, so happy – breathe out
I am breathing in – breathe in
I am breathing out – breathe out
In the here and in the now – breathe in and then out

Ask children when they can use their breathing. How about when we are really angry? Breathe! How about if we are bored and impatient in the grocery store with Mom? Breathe! What if we are really, really scared? Breathe! What if we are really, really excited? Breathe! Remind them to KNOW that they are breathing, and that they are sad, angry, scared, bored, etc.

Moon Breathing – good for full or new moon days

Either standing or sitting down, start in prayer position, *anjali mudra*. Inhale hands and arms up over head and tell children to imagine that they are the moon and that they are parting the heavens. Exhale as children extend arms and hands down to the sides as a circle, bringing all the stars and energy down around them and the earth. Then inhale and tell them to draw up the energy in the hands into the heart space again. Exhale hands to heart to end cycle in prayer position, *anjali mudra*. Repeat.

Balloon Breathing

Have children quiet themselves and imagine that they are a balloon. On the first breath in, they are getting ready to blow up a big balloon. On the exhale the balloon gets big. When they breathe in, the balloon deflates. Repeat. They can use their body as well. On the exhalation, move a leg or lift the arms.

Rag Doll Breathing

Begin standing in mountain pose, *tadasana*. Starting from the head and neck, children slowly with each breath begin to roll down the spine, letting arms hang loose as they move toward the floor. Tell them to go as slowly as possible, each breath just going down a little at a time. When they reach their toes, they can begin to breathe in again and roll up back to standing.

WARMUPS

Mountain Chant – *Tadasana*

Use this pose to begin all warmups. Return to this pose after finishing a warmup or transitioning into other poses

Standing steady in **mountain pose**. Feet fist–width apart and firmly planted, shoulders on the back, lower back full, neck lengthened, and arms steady at sides. Have children breathe and feel their feet in the earth. Have children repeat the chant back to you as you say it.

I am a mountain strong and steady
For everything now I am ready

Use affirmations. "I am strong! I am powerful!"

Polar Bear Chant – preschool – see appendix for music

Polar bear, polar bear,
Great big paws and great big jaw

Standing without moving feet, children swing arms, body and face side to side like a walking bear.

Walking on the ice and snow
Hunting for the fish in the water below

Bending at the waist with legs wide, ***prasarita padotanasana***, gentle swinging of one arm up, one arm down, windmills, twisting at the waist, then switching hands, as if they are fishing. Repeat.

Cheetah Chant – preschool – see appendix for music

Cheetah, cheetah, cheetah, running, running fast.
Cheetah, cheetah, cheetah, running through the grass.

Reaching and stretching up toward the ceiling with arms, left and then right. Ask children, "What is the cheetah chasing?"

Children can call out animals. Make animal sound. Then run in place.

Running, running, running, running!

Oh! It got away!

Repeat chant and question.

Kitty Cat Warmup – preschool and up

Start in **table pose**. There is a little cat, **cat cow pose**, playing with a ball of yarn. Thread right arm through opening between left arm and body and lie on arm. Twirl fingers around as if playing with ball of yarn. Repeat other side. A dog came along, **downward dog**, *adho mukha svanasana*, and scared kitty away. Bend knees, jump to **standing forward bend**, *uttanasana*. Inhale all the way back up to standing. Kitty cat goes out to play in the grass. Legs together, arms up overhead and fingers interlaced with index fingers pressed together to a point. Inhale up in the center, and then exhale over to the right. Inhale up to center, exhale over to the left. Repeat, and then exhale hands down and back into heart space.

Seashore Warmup

Sitting in crisscross applesauce, **lotus pose**, *padmasana*

You are a **lighthouse** — inhale at center, turn neck left and exhale. Return to center inhale, exhale turn neck to right — sending light to yourself and also out to everybody. There is a **seagull** on the shore — lift arms up above head and then down. Inhale raise the arms, exhale lower the arms. You get in a boat, **boat pose**, *navasana*. Create oars with your hands and fingers spread wide. Sing "row, row, row your boat." The **boat** begins to rock. Back to **lotus**, rock side to side with both hips on the ground. Inhale left arm up overhead and exhale, stretch to the right. Reverse sides. Rock the boat more. Sitting on tailbone, holding knees, rock forward and back slowly on spine and use tummy to pull back up again. Then have stronger and stronger waves as a storm hits, rocking back and forward on back of spine. Crash on shore, **sitting forward bend**, *paschimotanasana*. Then a **crab** walks by, *purvotanasana*. The crab pinches you to get up. Lifting up right leg while in crab pose, pinch with the toes. Switch left. Come to **standing forward bend**, *uttanasana*, inhale and bring arms and torso all the way up to standing, **mountain pose**, *tadasana*, and return to heart space, *anjali mudra*.

Spaceship Warmup

Sitting in **lotus pose**, *padmasana*. Shrug shoulders up, place on back, arms away from sides like a V and fingers pointing down. Breathing in and out to warm up the engine. Twisting torso and left arm in front and right arm in back to right, gently twisting and switching arms. Place hands on shoulders, make shoulder circles, getting ready for blast off, then stop and twist shoulders left to right again.

Inhale arms up over the head, hands interlaced and reaching toward the sky, exhale and blast off. Ask kids where in the world they want to go. Pluto! Inhale, then exhale and extend over to the right side and stretch. Inhale back and up and extend arms to other side. Bring arms down at sides again. Get out of your spaceship and into the rover. Press up into **crab pose**, *purvotanasana*. Head back, eyes roll around and around and look around. Exhale down to sitting again.

Ask another child where he wants to go. Jupiter (or Disneyland, grandma's house, etc.) Repeat so each child (or a few) gets a turn. Make suggestions for children who can't think of anything.

You've made your final landing. Get into **table position** and get into the space rover and do **cat cows** as it moves over bumpy terrain. Get out of the rover and explore by foot. **Runner's lunges**, both sides. Hide! Sit back on sit bones into **child's pose, *balasana***. What's there? An alien jumps out! **Lion pose, *simhasana***, roar loudly and open the eyes wide. Repeat three times.

Butterfly Warmup

Sit in **bound angle pose, *baddha konasana***, on floor. Explain that *mariposa* means butterfly in Spanish and that "*¿A donde vas?*" means "Where are you going?"

"*Mariposa, mariposa. ¿A donde vas?*"

Teacher calls on a child. Child names favorite place or where he wants to fly to. Lift up legs and knees, flying like a butterfly a few times. Then lengthen spine and stretch forward. Inhale back up again. Press back into **crab pose**, extend to *purvotanasana*. Repeat chant, picking another child in circle and so on.

Snake Warmup

Beginning in **child's pose, *balasana***, say to children:

¿Serpiente, serpiente, como estás?
Snake, snake, how are you?

Choose a child to respond.

Child moves into **cobra pose, *bhujangasana***, and says:

Bien, gracias.
I am well, thank you.

Have children hiss the sssss of *gracias* like a snake. Kneel back into **child's pose, *balasana***. Continue cycle of choosing another child. A child may be able to ask the question in Spanish as well.

Blooming Flower

Start in **standing forward bend, *uttanasana*.**

¿Florita florita, porque eres chiquita?
Little flower, little flower, Why are you so small?

Begin to grow by rolling up with the spine, slowly breathing in and out.

Crece, crece, crece.
Grow, grow, grow.

When children reach the hips, exhale. Inhale arms up at sides then reach arms all the way up above the head, reaching up high in the sky.

Florita, Florita, la vida es bonita.
Little flower, little flower, life is beautiful.

Let fingers dance around in the sunlight. Look up like a blooming flower. Interlace fingers together over head with index and thumb fingers together and pointing straight. Flower is blowing in the wind. Exhale and stretch to the left. Inhale back to center. Exhale over to right. Repeat three times.

Prize–Winning Warmup

Get ready to run a race! Start in **mountain pose, *tadasana*.** Inhale arms up then bow down into **forward standing bend, *uttanasana*.** Inhale half way up, exhale then step back with left leg into **runner's lunge.** Place back foot and come into **warrior I, *virabhadrasana I*.** Raise arms up over head. "I do my best. I know I can do it!" Step back up to ***uttanasana*.** Repeat other leg in **runner's lunge.** In one quick movement, switch to another **runner's lunge** on opposite leg. Stretch and repeat four times. On opposite leg, **runner's lunge** again. Raise arms up over head and give thanks to the audience. "I give thanks." Then ***uttanasana*,** inhale arms and torso up, claim your prize and bring hands into heart space.

Dog Show Warmup

We are at the dog show! Starting in **mountain pose, *tadasana*,** then **standing forward bend, *uttanasana*.** Step back into **downward dog, *adho mukha svanasana*.** Bend knees slightly. Have kids wiggle their bottoms like a tail, then straighten legs. Call out different types of dogs, such as sled dog, puppy dog, salty dog, hot dog, husky, etc. Ask children to call them out. In between each dog, bring a leg forward into **runner's lunge.** Then back to **downward dog** when one is called out. Be sure to switch each leg each time. Then come to **warrior pose I, *virabhadrasana I*,** and claim the prize. Switch sides.

Earth and Sky Warmup

Begin standing in **mountain pose,** *tadasana*. Hands in **heart position,** *anjali mudra*. Inhale arms up over head, exhale and bow forward. Inhale lengthen half way up, scoop up all the energy out of the earth and bring it inside you. Exhale, bow forward. On the next inhalation, bring your arms and body all the way back to upright position, arms up over the head, gather up all the energy in the sky, or heaven, or universe … and bring it into your heart. Exhale. Bring arms down and out to the sides, back to **heart position,** *anjali mudra.*

I AM Warmup

Begin standing in **mountain pose,** *tadasana*. Hands in **heart position,** *anjali mudra*. Turn palms away from face. Bring fingertips together and thumbs touching one another so that the hands form a triangle between them. Bring the hands down to the hip area. Say, "I am." Bring the hands into **heart position,** *anjali mudra,* and say, "I am Love." Bring hands and arms over head. Form a triangle with the index fingers coming together and the thumbs coming together and look up at it above your head. Say, "I am Light." Hands back into heart space. Inhale arms up over head, palms together, say, "I am heaven (or sky)." Exhale bow forward into **forward bend,** *uttanasana*. Say, "I am earth." Inhale, come all the way back up, hands together again, bring energy into heart and say, "I am."

Sun Salutation, *Surya Namaskar*

Include sun salutations in every class. I usually do three rounds. After the children have learned it, choose a child to lead it.

Have children repeat the chant back to you as you perform it.

1) Standing in **mountain pose,** *tadasana*, hands in heart space, *anjali madra*, breathing in.

2) Reach arms overhead. Exhale and bow down to

The sun the sun

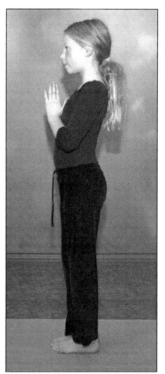

1)

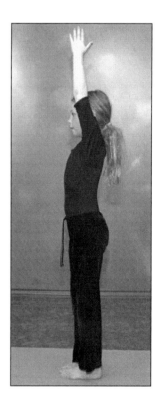

2)

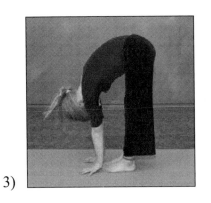

3)

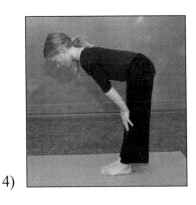

4)

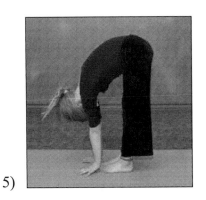

5)

3) **Standing forward bend,** *uttanasana.*

I salute the sun

4) Inhale halfway up.

I open my heart

5) Exhale back to **forward bend.**

to everyone

6) Inhale left leg back into **runner's lunge.**

The sun rises

7) Exhale right leg back into **plank pose.**

and the sun sets

8) Inhale lower knees down.

The whole world

9) Exhale lie on floor.

in my heart rests

6)

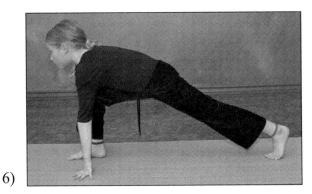

7)

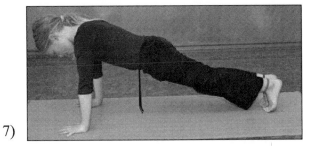

8)

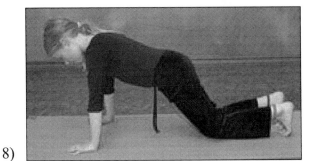

9)

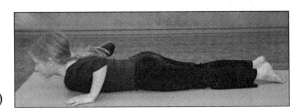

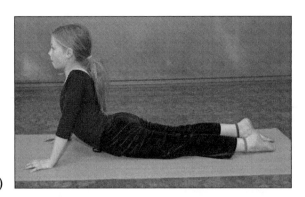

10)

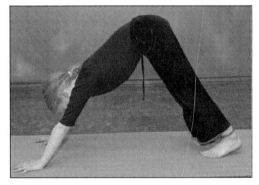

11)

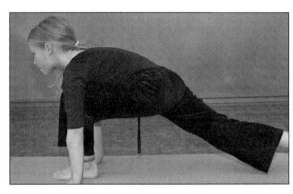

12)

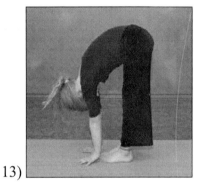

13)

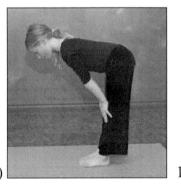

14)

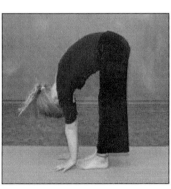

15)

10) Inhale up **cobra pose, *bhujangasana*.** Kids can hiss.

Again I arise

11) Exhale turn toes under, **downward dog,** ***adho mukha svanasana*.** Kids can bark.

ready to live

12) Inhale right leg forward in **runner's lunge** again.

happy to be

13) Exhale come to **standing forward bend,** ***uttanasana.***

and ready to give.

14) Inhale halfway up again.

The sun the sun

15) Exhale **forward bend.**

I salute the sun

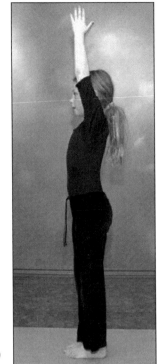

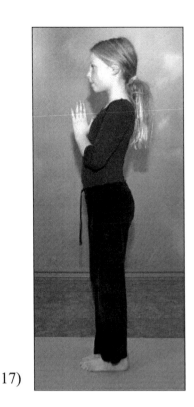

16)   17)

16) Inhale strong legs to pull arms and self all the way up over head. Kids like to give a clap when they come up with hands over head.

I open my heart

17) Exhale hands back into heart space.

to everyone.

After sun salutations, ask them to stand in **mountain pose**, *tadasana*, with their hands in ***an-jali mudra*** at their heart space. Have them close their eyes and ask them to notice how their body feels. Allow them to feel the energy in their bodies and allow any feelings to arise. Let them become aware of their feelings, energy, etc. Have them imagine the power of the sun inside them and that through their hands, feet, heart, etc., they are receiving love and peace and are sending their special gifts out to the world.

After several classes, many children will be able to lead a round of sun salutations.

SCRIPTED STORIES

USING SCRIPTED STORIES

Tell the following nine scripted stories by gathering the children around you. The bigger the class, the better to have them closer in a circle around you for the story. Before each story, discuss its geographical origin, if applicable. Ask, "Where is China, Egypt, England, etc.?" A simple blow–up globe or world–map placemat is helpful to illustrate this. When finished telling the story, tell the children, "Now help me retell the story with yoga!"

Perform the yoga poses and ask the children during the reenactment, "Who is the main character? Who is the hero? Who is the villain?" Continue going through the story asking, "What happens next? And then what happened? Who was at the well? What gifts did the snake give to the sailor?" Use images from the story to make questions. Lead the question's answer toward an asana. If you see the image of a tree in the story, ask a question that the tree symbol and asana (*vrksasana*) answers. For example, in *The Peddler's Dream*, ask, "What was next to the peddler's house? What was pushing up his house? A tree!"

This will also help prepare students for making up their own stories to add yoga poses to. If the children are having a hard time, as preschool children may have, prompt them by very briefly telling the story's sequence, recalling specific images and asking them questions about the story. Make funny faces and act out the pose to help them recall. You might have to tell the whole story, but even the youngest kids are really bright.

If you have time after *shavasana*, ask children to tell the story back to you. Choose three children who will tell the beginning, middle or end of the story. Ask each child to tell his part, then demonstrate to the class one asana he learned and can do at home, gym or at recess, etc.

After each class, tell children that they are all great yogis, and that they are all storytellers. Urge them to practice at home with their parents and to tell the story to them at dinnertime, story-time or any other time.

THE WARRIOR'S JOURNEY — original story by Sydney Solis
Theme: Yoga and You

This class is dedicated to welcoming each child to the lesson and to helping him or her become familiar with yoga, yoga poses, class and story structure. This story is acted out as it is told. You do not have to do all the poses and you may add any ones you like. Use affirmations freely.

You are the hero of your own story! **Warrior I, *virabhadrasana I*.** Take pose, both sides. You have a big heart and are kind!

You are going on a journey! "I believe in myself. I will succeed!"

Walking on the journey, you go this way — **triangle pose, *trikonasana*** — and that way, repeat **triangle pose** other side. You go up a hill — **side angle pose, *parshvakonasana*** — and down a hill — *parshvakonasana* — opposite side, arm comes down. Repeat sides.

You cross a bridge — **bridge pose, *setu banda sharvangasana*** — over a lovely river, bend at hips, straight back, arms out in front. You come to a tree — **tree pose, *vrksasana*.** Arms go up and flower. Do both sides.

You decide to rest. Coming down to floor — *janu shirsanasa* — leg stretch. Both sides, then spread both legs out — *uppavishta konasana*. Then you lie down and go to sleep — **hero's pose, *virasana*** — then lie all the way back — *supta virasana*.

All the animals are your friends. They come down a slide from a rainbow — *purvotanasana*. Into an **upward facing bow pose, *urdva dhanurasana*.** Many animals come and visit. Add as many animals as you wish. **Cobra pose, *bhujangasana*** (kids can hiss); dog — **downward dog pose, *adho mukha svanasana*** (bark); **camel pose, *ustrasana*; fish pose, *matsyasana*;** turtle — *kurmasana*; crow — *bakasana*; frog — *bekasana*; pigeon — *eka pada rajakapotanasana prep*.

The hero awakes and looks at all of creation — the animals, the earth, the body. You look this way — **seated twist pose, *ardha matsyendrasana I*.** He reflects on the heart and remembers where he came from.

The animals give you a present. It's a bow — **bow pose, *dhanurasana*** — and arrow — **warrior III, *virabhadrasana III*.** You thank the animals and say goodbye. But you are a new person — **feather dancer pose, *natarajasana*.**

Go across the bridge again — **floor bridge pose, *setu banda sharvangasana*.** Get into a boat near a beautiful lake — **boat pose, *navasana*.** Then get out of the boat, and go home, and reflect on the wonderful journey — **child's pose, *balasana*.** You are a different and better person because of your journey.

Discussion

Children are only too happy to express themselves. Encourage this by asking them how they feel afterwards, what pose they liked best and why. Explain that this is the journey of their selves and that they are the heroes of each story. Ask them to talk about something special about themselves or to name a thing they do especially well. Have a story stick or small object that can be passed around to each child, symbolizing that each has a turn to talk while others are quiet and listen. Tell a personal story about some journey that you took by yourself and how it changed you or how it made you feel. Get children to talk and tell stories about other journeys they have taken.

THE RABBIT IN THE MOON – India
Theme: Helping, sacrifice

Once far, far away, there lived a group of animals that were friends. There was a rabbit, a monkey, an elephant and an otter.

They lived in a beautiful, lush green forest with abundant mangos, bananas and papaya to eat. Above them a lovely moon shined and watched over them most nights.

All of the animals were very nice, but the rabbit was a very special creature. He seemed to radiate love and joy from his inner being. One day the rabbit called his friends together and said:

"My friends, every day we enjoy such bounty, I think it would be nice if we shared this with somebody who has less than we do. Let's share with the next person who comes through this forest."

The animals agreed. Now listening in on this was a great spirit. He was impressed by the rabbit's kindhearted gesture. He followed the animals around, listening.

The elephant said, "I will give the person a trunkful of cool water to drink."

The otter said, "I will dive into the stream and bring fish for the person to eat."

The monkey said, 'I'll climb up this tree and bring down some bananas to offer."

The rabbit began thinking. "My friends have so many wonderful things to offer that humans like. Rabbits eat grass and I do not think a human will like grass very much. Come to think of it, I have heard humans like rabbit meat. That's it! I will build a fire and give myself to the human to eat."

The great spirit heard this and was amazed. He decided to become a beggar man to test the rabbit and appeared the next morning.

"Look!" the animals all cried. "A human in the forest! Let's bring him our gifts!"

The animals all laid their gifts before the beggar man, who was really the great spirit. The beggar man thanked them.

It was the rabbit's turn to give his gift.

"I have nothing to give but myself," the rabbit said. He built a fire, lit it and leapt into the roaring flames. However, not a flame touched him. The beggar man reached with his hand into the fire and caught the rabbit, protecting him and lifting him out of the flames.

"You have done a great, fearless and unselfish thing. Everyone should always be able to see for themselves your great actions and example." So the beggar lifted the rabbit up, up, up high into the sky until he reached the moon, and that's where he rests.

People in India say that they see the rabbit in the moon. Look up at the next full moon and see if you can find the rabbit and remember the rabbit's example.

THE RABBIT IN THE MOON – yoga poses

The Hero — **warrior I,** *virabhadrasana I*

The Rabbit — **rabbit pose**. Also can jump like a rabbit.

The Elephant — elephant swings. Swing, standing, hands clasped together, stretched out front. Swing at waist left to right. Elephants are strong, so you can also do **warrior III,** *virabhadrasana III* or **warrior I,** *virabhadrasana I,* bring hands and index fingers together to a point for a trunk and extend upward.

The Otter — do **cat/cows** or from **table pose** lower hips to the floor with knees together left and then to the right.

The Monkey — **front splits,** *hanaumanasana*. Kids can jump like a monkey as well.

Tree — **tree pose,** *vrksasana*

Monkey getting mangoes — **camel pose,** *ustrasana*. Extend right arm up, left hand still on heel. Then switch.

Elephant getting water — **forward standing bend,** *uttanasana*. Then inhale torso and arms up, hands together, index fingers to a point. Then bend left and right.

Otter getting fish — **fish pose,** *matysanasana*

Rabbit in the fire — **bound angle pose,** *baddha konasana*

The Moon — **half moon pose,** *ardha chandrasana*

Lifting the rabbit to the moon — **moon breathing** in circles while sitting.

Discussion

Tell a story about how you helped somebody. For instance, did you help your mother do the dishes? Help your little sister tie her shoe? Is there something that you have done for yourself? Ask about ways that we can give. What does a favor mean? What nice things have been given to us? How do we feel when we receive? When we give? Is there anything that we had that was important to us and we gave it away? Anything great about ourselves that we would have to sacrifice in order to help another?

It's also a wonderful opportunity to talk about the moon. When was the last time you looked up at the moon, or studied its cycles? You'll be surprised what you see with a simple pair of binoculars. Encourage children to do the same.

THE PEDDLER'S DREAM — England
Theme: Following your dreams, believing in yourself

Once there was a man, a peddler, who lived in a house way out in the country. His house was a little cottage and next to it was a large apple tree. This tree's roots were so big that they were coming out of the ground and were beginning to push up one corner of the house. But the peddler didn't mind. He was very happy living in his house with his little dog.

One night, he had a dream. He dreamed that a voice said:

"Go to London Bridge. Go to London Bridge!"

That morning he woke up and said: "What a strange dream I had! A voice telling me to go to London Bridge! Well, London is so far away! I can't possibly make that journey." And he went about his business selling his wares in the town.

That night, he had the same dream.

"Go to London Bridge! Go to London Bridge!"

He thought how strange it was to have that dream again. But once again he ignored it.

The next night he had the exact same dream.

"Go to London Bridge! Go to London Bridge!"

It seemed to shout at him and he thought: "I can't stand it anymore. I must be crazy, but I'm going to London Bridge!"

So he said goodbye to his little dog and to his apple tree and set out down the road. He went this way, and that way. Up hills and down hills. He passed by donkeys and birds, and thought, "What a wonderful journey this is."

Finally he reached London and found London Bridge. What was he supposed to do now? he thought. He didn't know. So he sat, and he sat, and he sat. Nothing happened. He sat, and he sat, and he sat. Nothing happened. It began to get dark, so he lay down and slept.

The next morning he waited again. He sat, and he sat, and he sat. He sat, and he sat, and he sat. Finally, he said: "Oh, what a fool I've been! Following a dream! I'm wasting my time!" And he started to storm off.

Just then a man in a shop came running out after the peddler, crying, "Wait!" The peddler stopped. The shopkeeper said:

"Sir, I've seen you sitting here hour after hour for two days now. I've been wondering, what on earth are you doing? What are you waiting for?"

The peddler, somewhat embarrassed, said: "Well, to tell you the truth, I kept having this dream over and over again, night after night that said, 'Go to London Bridge! Go to London Bridge!' So finally I thought I'd do something about it. But this is all I got! Nothing!"

"Oh, yes! Dreams!" The shopkeeper laughed. "They are so silly. You know, many years ago I used to have a dream over and over again just like you. In the dream I dreamed that there was some house way out in the country with an apple tree whose roots were pushing up one side of the house! And beneath that apple tree was a treasure! Can you imagine? Me, going all the way out to the country looking for some silly apple tree? Dreams! That's all they are!"

But the peddler was thinking. He immediately said: "Goodbye! Thank you!" And he ran off, excited all the long way back to his house.

He dug under that apple tree. What do you think he found? Treasure! Diamonds, rubies, pearls! In his own back yard, by following and honoring his dream.

THE PEDDLER'S DREAM – yoga poses

Begin in **mountain pose, *tadasana*.**

The Peddler — **warrior I, *virabhadrasana I***

The tree at his house — **tree pose, *vrksasana***

Dog — **downward dog pose, *adho mukha svanasana***

Decides to go to London Bridge. Goes this way — **triangle pose, *trikonasana*** — and that way, opposite side.

He goes up a hill — **side angle pose, *parshvakonasana*** — and down a hill, both sides.

Passes by birds — **eagle pose, *garudasana***

And donkeys — kick like a donkey.

Arrives at London Bridge — **bridge pose, *setu bandha sarvangasana***

He sat, and he sat, and he sat — **chair pose, *utkatasana*** — three times

Goes down to rest — *janu shirsasana, uppavishta konasana*

Then goes to sleep — **hero pose, *virasana, supta virasana***

Next morning gets up. Sits and sits and sits again — **chair pose,** *utkatasana* — three times

Man comes out of the shop — **warrior II,** *virabhadrasana II*

Peddler stands in silence. He knows it's him!

Runs home — running in place

Digs up treasure — digging, swinging at waist and digging. Ask children what is in their treasure chest.

Treasure — **bound angle pose,** *baddha konasana*

Stand up, then bring treasure into the heart.

Diamonds — **twists ,** *ardha matyendrasana I*

Rubies — **bow pose,** *dhanurasana*

Pearls — **camel pose,** *ustrasana*

Discussion

What kinds of dreams do you have? Do you remember them? Encourage children to talk about and try and remember their dreams at night.

What do you want to be when you grow up? What dreams do you have for yourself, your friends and your family? When we honor our dreams they can be powerful guides to our life.

Encourage children to write down dreams in a little dream notebook and make up stories about the dreams. Also, they can make pictures or paintings or other creative expressions about dreams they've had.

THE LION'S WHISKER – Somalia and Sudan
Theme: Patience, persistence

There was once a woman who married a widower with a son. His son was a fine young man, and the woman loved him and wanted to make him like her own son. But when she tried to hug him, he resisted.

"Go away! You are not my real mother!" he said. "My real mother is dead! I hate you!"

The woman was so sad. She tried everything to make him love her. She made his favorite meals. But the boy just threw them at her! She tried talking to him, but he stomped away furious.

She was so unhappy that she decided to consult a witch doctor who was famous for making love potions.

"I want you to make me a love potion so that my stepson will love me!" she said to the doctor.

"That is a very difficult thing to do," the doctor said.

"I'll do anything!" the woman cried.

"Well, you must first bring me the whisker of a lion," the doctor said.

"The whisker of a lion? How on earth am I going to do that?" she said. "How do you approach a ferocious lion?"

"I require the whisker of a lion if you wish to make the love potion," the doctor said. "I told you it would be difficult."

The woman was determined to make her stepson love her, so she devised a plan. One moonlit night, she took all of the courage she had inside her and went deep into the jungle looking for a lion. As she crawled through the jungle, strange birds passed by her and snakes crawled in front of her. But she was determined.

She came to a cave. There inside it slept a great lion. The woman had brought some food with her. She put the food down and backed away.

The lion woke up and roared. Then he saw the food and gobbled it up.

The next morning the woman came again. This time she got a little closer before leaving the food for the lion. Then she snuck away. The lion roared again, and gobbled everything up. She did this for many days, until one day, she put the food so close to the lion and he was so used to her that he let her get right next to him. She stroked his soft hair and the lion purred in happiness. Very quickly she plucked a whisker out of his face. Overjoyed, she ran all the way to the witch doctor and showed him the whisker.

"Look! I have the lion's whisker! Now make the love potion!"

The witch doctor took the whisker and examined it closely. He then threw it in the fire before them and it burned up immediately with a hiss and a puff.

"How could you have done that?" the woman screamed, looking horrified. "You don't know what I went through and how long it took me to get that lion to trust me!"

"If you were able to give that kind of patience to earn a lion's trust, then surely you can have that patience to earn your stepson's trust," the witch doctor said.

The woman suddenly understood and went home to her stepson. She was loving and patient with him, and in time the stepson grew to love his stepmother.

THE LION'S WHISKER – yoga poses

The mother — **warrior I, *virabhadrasana I*** — both sides

The son — he is firm in his stance toward his mother — **mountain pose, *tadasana***

Told her to go away — moon breathing arm circles

Witch doctor — **warrior II, *virabhadrasana II***

Journey into the jungle — **side angle pose, *parshvakonasana*** — both sides

Crawls on the jungle floor — **pigeon pose, *eka pada rajakapotanasana prep*** — both sides

Sees snake on the path — **cobra pose, *bhujangasana***

Sees birds on the path — **eagle pose, *garudasana***

Return to floor with **forward standing bend, *uttanasana***. Step legs back into **plank pose,** lower all the way down.

Woman leaves food — stretch arms out in front then press back into **child's pose, *balasana***.

Affirmations: "I am patient! I am calm! I can do it!"

Lion roars — **lion pose, *simhasana***

Have children eat up the food. Ask the kids what kind of food it is and to animate eating it.

Lion rests back in **child's pose,** *balasana.*

Next day mother comes again — **runner's lunges** — left and right

Repeat lion roar, eating up food, then **child's pose.**

Last time — she puts the food down. Lies back in **hero's pose,** *supta virasana,* to wait as lion is nice this time and eats up the food. Woman gets closer, lying on stomach — **upward facing boat pose,** *purna navasana* — plucks off the lion's whisker. Have kids act out plucking off a whisker.

Goes back to the magician and she's so happy she's going to roll home — **bow pose,** *dhanurasana* — have children rock over to left side and then right.

Gives whisker to the witch doctor, and he burns it up. Release from **bow pose,** collapse. She can't believe this happened.

But when she understands the witch doctor's words, she understands and her heart opens — **camel pose,** *ustrasana.*

Discussion

Have children talk about a time in their lives when they were patient. What did they do? What happened? For younger children give suggestions. For example: Did you wait in line? Did you wait your turn to play? Older kids can give more detailed stories.

Tell a personal story about something you accomplished that was difficult to do.

Remind children that when faced with difficulty or impatience, they can breathe, or do the breathing song to relax and remain calm and peaceful.

THE MAGIC PEAR TREE – China
Theme: Non–greed, giving

Once there was a very old man who wandered into a small village in China. He had nothing but the clothes on his back and the shoes on his feet. The people immediately knew who he was and were not afraid of him. He was a wandering monk, and the people liked him. They knew that these wandering monks could do magic.

Every day the monk begged for his food and the people gladly gave him some rice or vegetables.

"Don't beg from Farmer Chu," a little boy warned him. "He never gives anything to anyone. He will drive you away!" The old man thanked the boy for the advice.

One morning there was a festival in the market and all the people gathered there. Farmer Chu came, too. He had a huge wooden cart filled with pears that was pulled by a donkey. He was cruel to the donkey, whipping it and yelling at it to make it move faster. It was very hot that day, so people bought farmer Chu's pears even though he was so mean, because the pears were so sweet and juicy and satisfied their thirst.

The old man decided to ask Farmer Chu for a pear.

"Get away from me you old beggar man! You're not getting anything from me!" Farmer Chu shouted.

People yelled at Farmer Chu, "Give the old man a pear, you stingy fool." But Farmer Chu refused. Finally, a woman bought the old man a pear.

The old man thanked her, held it up and said, "Everyone, you have been so kind to me and gave me food to eat. I wish to give something back to you."

Everyone gathered around. The old man ate the pear slowly and enjoyed every bite. He then saved one small, black seed. He put the seed in the ground, then asked a boy to go fetch a kettle of boiling water. The boy brought the water and the old man poured it onto the seed.

Instantly the seed began to sprout before their very eyes. The people watched in amazement as the sprout grew and grew and soon became an enormous pear tree. The tree flowered and soon pears appeared, ripe and ready to eat!

The old man climbed up, picked the pears and passed them out to everyone. The pear tree then began to wither and soon died. The old man set about chopping it down, and magically, he had enough firewood to give out to everybody. The people thanked the old man. He bowed deeply back to them and then slowly made his way out of town.

Just then, a shout was heard from the crowd.

"Stop thief! That man stole my pears!" It was Farmer Chu. He was standing where his cart used to be. There was nothing but his donkey and a wheel.

Everybody started laughing. They knew that the old man taught Farmer Chu a lesson. He used his magic to conjure away the farmer's pears and used the wood from his cart for the tree.

From then on people always said: "Don't be greedy, or you'll end up a fool like Farmer Chu!"

THE MAGIC PEAR TREE – yoga poses

The Old Man — **warrior I, *virabhadrasana I*** — begging for food — extend hands out

Little Boy — **warrior II, *virabhadrasana* II** — or — **side angle pose, *parkvakonasana***

Farmer Chu — come down to a squat, his heart is closed off — **demon pose.**

Go away — come back to standing on tiptoes. Moon breathing arm circles.

Pear — **camel pose, *ustrasana***

Planting the seed — ***prasarita padotanasana*** — legs stretched wide. Right hand comes down, left hand comes up into a twist. Twist at the navel. Plant the pear seed. Switch. Left hand comes down, right hand rises in the air. Repeat.

Hands on hips, shoulders on the back. Inhale and come up to standing.

Tea Pot — **feather dancer pose, *natarajasana*** — pouring the water on the seed. Both sides.

Tree — **tree pose, *vrksasana***. The tree flowers. Open arms up wide then gently bring down to sides.

Chopping down the tree. Inhale up and down. Bend at the waist.

Tree branches — ***janu sirsasana*** — both sides.

Bundles of firewood — **bound angle pose, *baddha konasana***

Donkey and Wheel — **donkey kicks** — and — **upward facing bow pose, *urdva dhanurasana***

Come to **downward dog, *adho mukha svinasana***. Jump to front of mat to **forward standing bend**, *uttanasana*, inhale and come up. Arms to heart space.

He stole my pears!

Laugh! Swing arms and body side to side. Roll on the floor.

Discussion

Ask children if there is anything that they remember giving away to somebody else. How did it make them feel? Can they remember a time when they didn't want to give something away? Why didn't they want to give it away? How did it make them feel? Tell a personal story about a time you had something you really liked but somebody else needed or wanted and you gave it to them. Ask children what kinds of things we can do to help the less fortunate, such as donate old toys, hold a bake sale and raise money for the homeless.

DIAMONDS, RUBIES AND PEARLS – Germany
Theme: Our actions matter

Once there was a lovely young girl who lived with her poor mother. One day her mother told her, "Daughter, please go up the hill and fetch me some water."

"Of course, mother." And she went up the hill.

When she got there, there was an old, old woman sitting by the well.

"Please young lady," the old woman asked. "I am so thirsty, won't you give me a drink of water?"

"Yes, of course! I'd be happy to. You just sit right down there and rest," the girl said.

The girl drew up the water from the well, then gave the old lady a drink.

"Thank you so much," the old woman said. "Because of your kindness, good luck will always be with you. Nothing but diamonds and rubies and pearls will come from your lips when you speak."

"What are you talking about?" the girl asked. Instantly, beautiful diamonds, rubies and pearls poured out of her mouth. A huge sparking pile now lay in front of her. The girl ran all the way back home yelling, and a glittering trail of jewels was left behind her.

When she came home she told her mother everything that had happened, and as she did another round of precious jewels poured out from her mouth.

Now, a neighbor was visiting the old lady at the time, and she saw what had happened and thought, "Well, if her daughter can get the jewels, my daughter certainly can, too. Maybe she can even get twice as many."

So she sent her daughter up the hill to get some water. And at the top of the hill the old, old woman was waiting there. The old, old woman asked her for some water.

"Go away, you ugly, old woman," the daughter said. "Stop bothering me. I'm not going to help you ever!" And she went to get her own water.

"Bad luck will always be with you," the old woman said. "Nothing but snakes and lizards and toads will come from your lips when you speak."

"What did you say?" the girl asked. Sure enough, snakes and lizards and toads poured out of her mouth. The girl dropped the bucket of water and ran all the way back down the hill screaming, a trail of snakes and lizards and toads behind her.

DIAMONDS, RUBIES AND PEARLS – yoga poses

The young girl — **warrior I,** *virabhadrasana I*

Her mother — **warrior II ,** *virabhadrasana II*

Going to get water — **triangle,** *trikonasana* — both sides

Going up the hill — **side angle pose,** *parshvakonasana* — both sides

Old woman — **warrior III,** *virabhadrasana III* — bring leg down to sides then bring arms and hands back to heart position

Well — *prasarita padotanasana* — then windmills

Drawing up the water — hands on hips, shoulders on the back, come up

Diamonds — **feather dancer pose,** *natarajasana*

Rubies — **camel pose,** *ustrasana*

Pearls — **upward facing bow,** *urdva dhanurasana* — or — **bridge pose,** *setu bandha sharvangasana*

Mean girl — **forward standing bend,** *uttanasana* — to a squat, heart closed off

Snakes — **snake pose,** *bhujangasana*

Toads — **frog pose,** *bekasana*

Lizards — *marichianasana II* — or — **upward facing dog pose,** *urdva mukha svinasana*

Discussion

Talk about how our words have power and can either do good or harm. How do our actions matter? Tell a story about a time when somebody hurt your feelings. What did they do? How did you feel? Talk about how caring for others is really taking care of ourselves.

GANESHA'S LESSON – India
Theme: Kindness, non–violence

One day the elephant–headed little boy–god named Ganesha went off to play in the woods of Mount Kailasa where he lived. He was a mischievous little boy and he especially loved to run and play and pretend that he was a warrior.

One day he took out his play bow and arrows.

"What can I hunt?" he thought. He spotted his little white cat and immediately pursued it. He shot his little arrows at the cat, and the cat ran off terrified. But Ganesha thought that the cat was having fun. So Ganesha searched for it and found the little cat shaking in fear behind a tree.

"Aha! I found you," he cried, and again shot arrows at the cat. But the little cat, still terrified, ran off. Once again Ganesha found the cat under a log and this time he pounced on the cat, rubbed its little body into the dirt, then threw it up in the air. But the cat ran off and Ganesha couldn't find it again.

"Well," Ganesha said. "This is no fun." And he went back home.

When he got there, he saw his mother, the Goddess Parvati. He stopped in his tracks when he saw that she had mud stains on her face and hands and scratches on her arms.

"Mother, what happened to you?" he asked.

Parvati looked at herself and said: "I don't know. Did you do this to me?"

"ME?" Ganesha exclaimed. "Why NO!" But just then, he looked down at his feet and said, "Oh, but you know what? I was rather rough with our cat today."

"Oh," his mother said, gathering him up in her arms. "Now I understand. You know, Ganesha, I am this whole world. My body is this whole earth. Anytime you do anything to it, you hurt me. You see, I was that little cat, too. So anything you did to it, you did to me.

"Oh, I understand now. My actions really do matter. I am so sorry, mother. I won't do it again."

"It's impossible not to do any harm to everything, but we can be very aware of our actions, so that we do as little harm as possible."

Ganesha thanked his mother for his lesson and went off to play again with the little cat, but without his bow and arrows.

GANESHA'S LESSON – yoga poses

Ganesha — elephant swings, **warrior I,** *virabhadrasana I* — bring hands and index fingers together to a point for a trunk and extend upward.

Mountain — **mountain pose,** *tadasana*

Cat — **cat, cow pose**

Trees — **tree pose,** *vrksasana*

Chasing the cat — **side angle pose,** *parshvakonasana* — and — **triangle pose,** *trikonasana* — or for little kids — running in place.

Bow — **bow pose,** *dhanurasana* — or left leg back, right foot forward, hips squared to front. Inhale arms up overhead and bring index fingers together at a point. Gently arch back like a bow.

Arrow — **warrior III,** *virabhadrasana III*

Mother Parvati — **warrior II,** *virabhadrasana II*

Gathering into lap — **bound angle pose,** *badha konasana*

Rocking in lap — take right leg and press right foot into left hand. Hold right knee inside right elbow. Then cradle foot into left elbow and rock like a baby. Repeat other side.

Run off to play again — **bow pose,** *dhanurasana* — then roll side to side.

Discussion

How can we be aware of our actions? How do we know the effect we have on others?

Give examples of cause and effect. If you run a red stoplight, what happens? If you pick a fight with somebody instead of making peace, what happens?

How do we do things to harm ourselves, such as negative thinking, poor choices, etc.? How can we treat ourselves kindly without harsh judgment? Tell a personal story about how your actions had a good or bad result, or how you have hurt yourself in the past.

THE BUFFALO DANCE – Native America
Theme: Respect, keeping promises

There was once a lovely young lady who woke up early one morning and went walking. She came to a cliff and saw all the buffalo at the edge. Her tribe considered the buffalo sacred and also depended on them for meat. So she cried out to the buffalo: "Please, buffalo, throw yourselves over the cliff so that you can give yourselves to us. If you do, I will marry one of you!"

Well, the buffalo heard her and they jumped over the cliff and became meat for her people. However, the head buffalo came up to her and said, "Now you and I will be married!"

"Oh, no!" she thought, but the buffalo reminded her of her promise. She knew she had to marry him. So she went off with the head buffalo. A beautiful magpie circled around the girl and called to her, then flew back to her people.

Back home, the young lady's father began to worry about his daughter. Where has she gone? He saw all the buffalo at the bottom of the cliff and was worried. The buffalo have her! The magpie swooped over the father and showed him where she was. When the girl went to get some water, she saw her father.

"Father! You must leave at once! This is too dangerous for you to be here!" And she went back to the buffalo. But the buffalo smelled something funny on her.

"Ah! I smell another human!" the buffalo cried. He found the father and trampled him. The girl was overwhelmed with grief and sadness and cried torrents of tears for her father. Now the buffalo was worried. He knew the humans had special magic. So he said,

"If you can bring your father back to life I will let you both leave."

So the girl asked the magpie to find a piece of her father. It brought back a piece of his backbone, which she covered with a blanket.

"Father, father, one, two, three. Father, father, return to me." And she danced in a circle. Her father returned to life.

The big buffalo thought this was amazing. He said: "If you can do this for your father, please do it for us. We give ourselves to you willingly to eat and use, but bring us back to life. I will teach you our dance."

And the buffalo taught her his dance, as well. "Buffalo, buffalo, one, two, three. Buffalo, buffalo, return to me." And they danced and danced.

So that is what the people do after the buffalo hunt. They respect and honor the buffalo and thank them for giving so much food, clothing and many other uses. And the buffalo were always plentiful.

THE BUFFALO DANCE – yoga poses

The Young Girl — **warrior I,** *virabhadrasana I*

The Buffalo — **downward dog,** *adho mukha svanasana* — children can paw the ground with their feet, lifting each leg up and down, then switching. Or any **warrior pose.**

Buffalo jumping over cliff — bow to **forward bend,** *uttanasana.* Staying in **forward bend,** do **standing splits** — lift one leg up, then bring down. Repeat both sides. Or — **chair pose,** *utkatasana* — and spring up from the pose each time as if jumping over a cliff.

The Father — **warrior II,** *virabhadrasana II*

The Magpie — **eagle pose,** *garudasana*

Girl goes to get water — *prasarita padotanasana* — **windmills**

Sad at her father's death — **reclining hero pose,** *supta virasana*

Piece of bone from father — **head to knee pose,** *janu shirsasana* — both sides.

Cover with blanket — **standing forward bend,** *uttanasana* — then step back into **plank pose,** lower down to floor — **upward facing bow pose,** *urdva navasana.*

Dance for father — children chant song. "Father, father, one, two, three. Father, father, return to me." While moving in a circle to the right, leaping onto each mat. Lift arms in the air and sway back and forth. Reverse sides and repeat.

Dance for buffalo — repeat dancing as above for father, but say, "Buffalo, buffalo, one, two three. Buffalo, buffalo, return to me."

Discussion

Ask children what kinds of things are they thankful for — food, clothes, toys? Ask them to think about where these items came from. What kinds of things had to happen so that the children could have and enjoy the items? Such as sun, earth and rain growing food. People sewing toys, etc.

How can we show these things respect and thanks? Discuss the ritual of saying grace before meals, taking care of our things and treating them well. What does it mean to take something for granted? Native Americans believed that if you don't thank something, it will go away. Was there ever a time when you didn't treat something nicely or give thanks?

Also discuss keeping our promises. Why is it important to keep our promises? What does it mean to be an honorable person? What kinds of promises did you make? What promises have you kept? Have you ever broken a promise?

THE SHIPWRECKED SAILOR – Egypt
Theme: Hope, courage, compassion

Once upon a time, a long, long time ago in ancient Egypt, there was a Captain of a ship. He had been lost at sea and lost his ship and everything it was carrying. He was very sad and worried he would get into trouble. Another Captain heard his story and said:

"Fear not, let me tell you a story. Once I was riding on a great ship. We had the strongest and most courageous men aboard. Their hearts were as fierce as lions. However, a terrible storm swept up and the ship was lost. I floated alone on a piece of wood from the ship, until I washed up on an island. There I found many trees with abundant food to eat, coconuts, figs and fish. I was so grateful, I made a fire and thanked the Gods.

"Just then, lightening struck and the ground shook and suddenly before me was a snake! It cried out, 'Who are you? Why have you come?'

"Quickly I told him everything that had happened to me.

"'Ah,' the snake said. 'I hear your cries. I, too, have lost things dear to me. A star once fell on this island and my whole family was lost. I was so sad. You and I, we are both survivors!'

"Just then, I thought of my own family and was sad, but he said:

"'Don't be afraid or be sad! Have courage! Good will come from your difficulty. You are safe here. And in four months, you will be rescued. A ship will come for you and you will see your family again!'

"I was so grateful! I told the serpent that I would send gifts of gold and many riches for his kindness and hospitality. But the serpent only laughed.

"'I have all the riches I could ever need! Besides, this island will disappear forever under the waves once you leave. But it will always be with you inside your heart. Whenever you have difficulty, have courage and remember the island that lives inside of you.'

"Indeed the serpent was right! A ship did come for me! I thanked the serpent and said farewell. The serpent asked that I say good things about him upon my return. He gave me many gifts, such as monkeys, dogs and many precious things, which I gave to the Pharaoh, who gave me a lovely house and made me lieutenant.

"So my friend," the Captain said to the other Captain. "Don't worry. And never fear. You never know what good comes from hardship."

THE SHIPWRECKED SAILOR – yoga poses

The Sailor — **warrior II,** *virabhadrasana II.*

Hearts as fierce as lions — **lion pose,** *simhasana.*

Boat — **boat pose,** *navasana.*

Island — **downward dog,** *adho mukha svanasana*

Tree — **tree pose,** *vrksasana*

Fish to eat — **fish pose,** *matsyasana*

Fire — **bound angle pose,** *baddha konasana*

Lightning — **warrior III,** *virabhadrasana III*

Serpent — **cobra pose,** *bhujangasana*

Star — **half-moon pose,** *ardha chandrasana*

Monkeys — jumping like a monkey — or — **splits,** *hanumanasana* — or — **side leg pose,** *janu shirsasana*

Dogs — **downward dog,** *adho mukha svanasana*

Remember the island that is always inside the heart — **camel pose,** *ustrasana*

Discussion

Ask children to talk about a time when they were scared. What happened? Who was there? How did they overcome their fear? Was there anything good that happened out of the difficulty?

Think of somebody who has had a hard time or problem. Ask children to relate similarities in their life to what happened to that person. How can we help others who are in distress?

POSES, *ASANAS*

There are many yoga poses out there, more than I can possibly put in this little book! But here are many of the basic poses used in this book. Children will vary greatly in their flexibility and ability to perform the poses. Always see the beauty in the child's original pose and effort and honor that, while directing the child into the full alignment of the pose. Introduce adjustments with the attitude of moving toward something in process, while we celebrate and rejoice in the present and our practice of yoga and completely accept and love our current situation.

You will find a lot of hyper–extended elbows and knees, wobbly legs, etc. But that's OK! Guide children into discovering their bodies. In time and practice they will improve. For ideas on more poses, consult B.K.S. Iygengar's classic, *Light On Yoga*.

BOAT POSE
Navasana

Begin seated with knees bent. Bring arms out straight in front near knees. Use stomach muscles to draw legs in and up. Extend legs out for full position.

Benefits

Strengthens abdominals. Improves digestion. Tones kidneys.

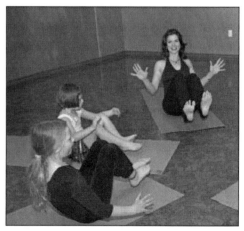
Boat Pose

What it looks like

A boat with oars, the letter V, a bowl of soup, a train.

BOUND ANGLE POSE
Baddha Konasana

Seated, bring feet together. Press feet together energetically, then extend out through the knees. Bow forward.

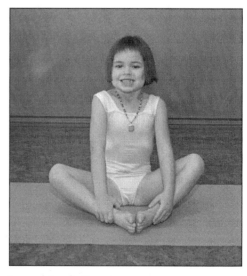
Bound Angle Pose

Benefits

Aids lower abdominal organs in functioning. Good for hip and knee joints. Helps with bladder control.

What it looks like

A butterfly, a plant, a flower pot.

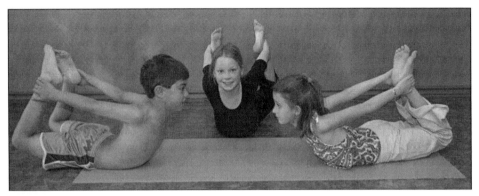

Bow Pose

BOW POSE
Dhanurasana

Begin lying face down. Bend knees. Bring shoulders on the back and grab ankles. Tuck the tailbone and arch up. Rock side to side for variation.

Benefits

Stretches the spine and keeps it flexible. Tones the abdominal organs

What it looks like

A bow, a circle, a bug, a ship.

BRIDGE POSE
Setu bandha sharvangasana

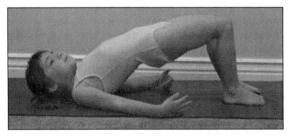

Bridge Pose

Begin lying on back. Bend knees and bring feet toward buttocks. Press hips up. Walk shoulder blades underneath and then clasp hands. Not all children will be able to clasp hands. Keep inner thighs moving toward each other and tuck the tailbone.

Benefits

Opens the chest and upper back. Develops the buttocks.

CAMEL POSE
Ustrasana

Kneeling with toes curved under or flat on the floor, place hands on hips. Extend and lift the spine as you arch the back. Drop the hands back onto the heels, press the hips forward, tuck tailbone.

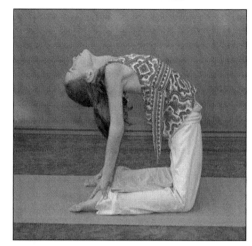

Camel Pose

Benefits

Develops hamstrings and inner thighs. Calms the mind and removes fatigue. Removes stiffness in neck and shoulders.

What it looks like

A tunnel, a mountain, going down a well to fetch water, any pose when a heart–opening realization occurs.

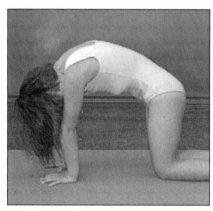

Cat Pose

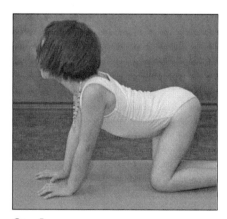

Cow Pose

CAT/COW POSE

Beginning in **table pose**, inhale. Exhale and arch back up like a cat. Inhale again and drop down like a cow.

Benefits

Good for the spine. Develops the wrists and arms.

What it looks like

A cat, a cow, a moving vehicle, a bumpy road, a bicycle pump, waves.

CHAIR POSE

Utakatasana

Begin in **mountain pose**. Raise arms over head, bend knees and bring together and sit as if sitting in a chair.

Benefits

Strengthens ankles, calves, inner thighs, back. Stretches the shoulders.

What it looks like

A princess with a puffy dress, a chair, a lightening bolt.

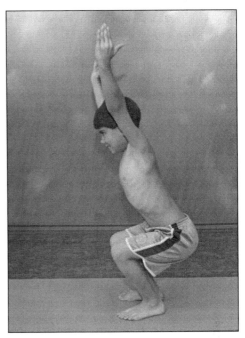

Chair Pose

CHILD'S POSE

Balasana

Have child spread knees and extend arms forward in front of them. Also may move arms to the sides.

Benefits

A good resting pose. Good for the lower back.

What it looks like

A ball, somebody praying, begging, sleeping.

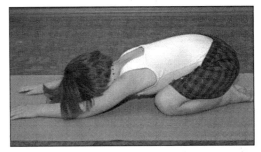

Child's Pose

COBRA POSE
Bhujangasana

Begin lying flat on stomach, hands back by the base of the breastbone. Uncurl toes and press into floor. Bring energy to the legs. Inhale up, shoulders on the back. Hiss like a snake.

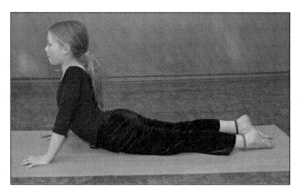

Cobra Pose

Benefits

Good for strengthening the back and spine. Expands the chest.

What it looks like

A snake, a piece of rope, a walrus.

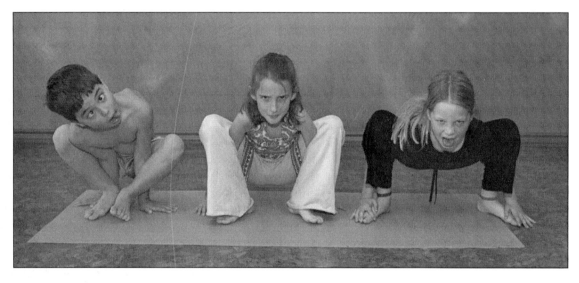

Demon Pose

DEMON POSE
Bhujapidasana

Come into a squat and place the hands on top of the feet. For variation, place hands on floor, shrug the shoulders and melt the heart. Keep the arms and hands strong as you squeeze with the inner thighs and lift off, balancing on the hands.

Benefits

Strengthens hands and wrists. Creates strong abdominals. Develops the leg and arm muscles.

What it looks like

Good for antagonist characters, demons, dragons, silly or scary creatures, tricksters.

DOWNWARD DOG POSE
Adho Mukha Shvanasana

Begin in **table pose**. Lean back toward heels, then press hips and buttocks up and back. Straighten legs.

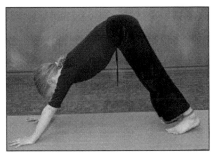

Downward Dog Pose

Benefits

Removes fatigue. Develops the ankles, arms and abdominals. Strengthens and relieves stiffness in shoulders. Good for digestion.

What it looks like

A tunnel, a mountain, a house, a dog stretching, an upside down V, a magic portal.

EAGLE POSE
Garudasana

Begin standing in **mountain pose, *tadasana***. Entwine left leg over the right leg. Extend left arm out, then cross right arm over it. Bend the elbows and entwine the two together and bring hands together. Release and fly out like an eagle. Reverse sides.

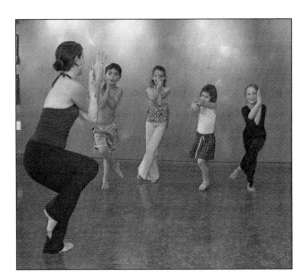

Eagle Pose

Benefits

Strengthens ankles. Stretches the shoulders. Removes cramps in calves.

What it looks like

A bird flying, twisted noodles.

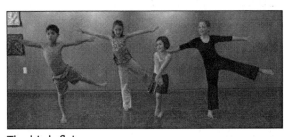

The birds fly!

EXTENDED LEGS POSE
Prasarita Padottanasana

Spread legs wide, feet and toes pointing forward. Bend forward, palms down on the floor. Can do "windmills" with one hand on the floor and the other extended, twisting from the navel area.

Benefits

Develops hamstrings and inner thighs. Calms the mind and removes fatigue.

What it looks like

A tunnel, a mountain, going down a well to fetch water, a windmill.

FEATHER DANCER POSE
Natarajasana

Begin standing on one leg and bring knee to hands. Bring right hand to hold right big toe. Then arch back and tuck tailbone. Press foot into hand. Extend left hand out and bow forward, balance. Reverse sides.

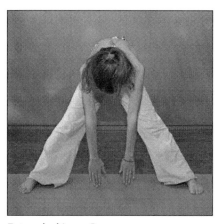

Extended Legs Pose

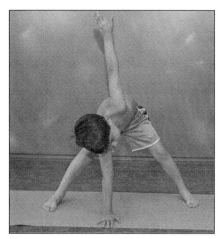

Windmill

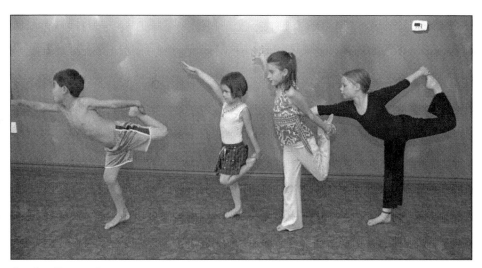

Feather Dancer Pose

Benefits

Strengthens leg muscles. Develops poise. Stretches the shoulders and expands the chest. Benefits the spine.

What it looks like

A dancer, a tea pot, a lightening bolt, a hunter, a gazelle.

FISH POSE
Matsyasana

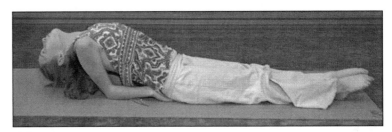

Fish Pose

Sit on hands, preferably palms facing down. Legs are extended. Drop elbows down to floor and arch back. Slide back enough so that head will touch the floor.

Benefits

Good for the abdominal organs.

What it looks like

A fish, a sleeping mermaid.

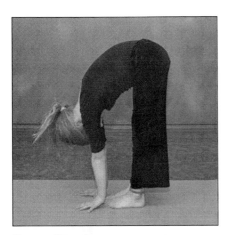

Forward Bend

FORWARD BEND
Uttanasana

Feet fist–width apart, bending over at the hips and hands touching the floor. Make feet, ankles, knees and legs strong.

Benefits

Good for concentration, removing fatigue. Good for stomach, liver, kidneys and heart. Stretches the hamstrings.

What it looks like

A folding chair, a sleeping praying mantis.

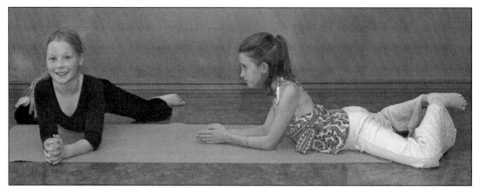

Frog Pose

FROG POSE
Bekasana

Begin in **table position**. Spread knees out toward edges of mat and bring heels together. Bow forward onto stomach and elbows. Press feet into each other and extend out through the knees.

Variation: Lower legs are perpendicular to upper legs and feet out.

Benefits

Abdominal organs are toned. Stretches the hips and thighs.

What it looks like

A frog, a diamond, a minnow, a swimmer under the deep sea.

HALF–MOON POSE
Ardha chandrasana

From **triangle pose**, bend right knee and take a small step with left foot. Balance on right foot, extend left leg out. Right hand is on the floor, left hand extends upward. Try looking at fingertips.

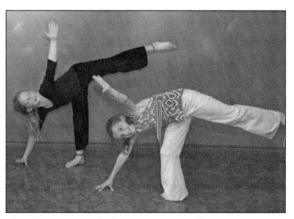

Half–Moon Pose

Benefits

Good for legs and lower spine. Strengthens core. Develops balance. Opens pelvis.

What it looks like

A moon, a wheel, a merry go round, scissors.

HANDSTANDS

Kids love to do handstands! Emphasize that this is NOT a HEADSTAND. These poses give kids confidence to do something that they usually don't do and the confidence to be in a situation where things may be turned upside down.

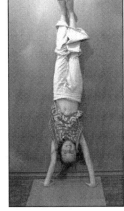

Start with an L handstand. They won't be able to be at an L, and their legs will be high on the wall. Over time their arms, tummies and legs will build up strength.

For regular handstands, children usually can't get themselves up. Big kids can kick up, or may need assistance. Little ones I assist, and just plain pick up their legs and hold them with their hands giving support.

HANDSTAND
Adho Mukha Vriksasana

Handstand

Begin in **table position** facing the wall. Shrug shoulders up and melt the heart. Keeping arms strong and shoulders on the back, press up into **downward dog**. From **downward dog**, take a step forward with and kick up with the back leg. Squeeze in with the inner thighs and extend feet up into the air.

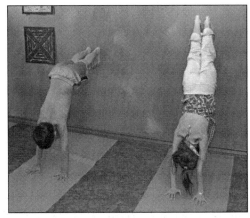

BENEFITS

Strengthens shoulders, arms and wrists. Expands the chest. Tones the organs.

L–HANDSTAND

L–Handstand

Begin seated with back against the wall, legs extended straight out. Let hands reach where heels were. Place hands, come into **table position**, then into **downward dog**. Step up with one foot against the wall, then press the other into the wall, both together.

HERO POSE
Virasana and Supta Virasana

Begin by kneeling. Bring legs and feet slightly out to the side of the leg, toes pointing straight back, then gently sit back as far as comfortable. Make ankles and toes active.

Benefits

Removes fatigue. Stretches quads and thighs. Relieves stomach problems. Calms the mind. Encourages deep breathing and a rested heart. Good for the knees. Opens the chest.

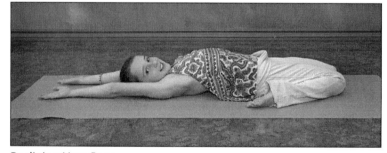

Hero Pose

What it looks like

Somebody who is tired and wants to take a nap, a frog king, a smiling fish, a heart.

Reclining Hero Pose

LION POSE
Simhasana

Start in **child's pose**, *balasana*, with arms and hands extended. Then press forward and let face go wild. Squish it up. Roar like a lion!

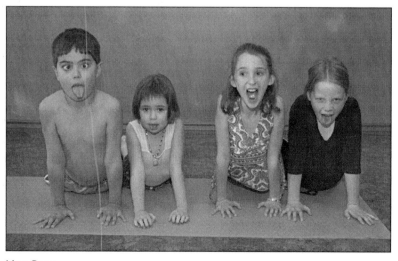

Lion Pose

Benefits

Good for the speech and stammers. Releases tension in the face, jaw and body. Revives expression.

What it looks like

A lion, an alien, monsters, giant squids, dragons, witches.

LOTUS POSE
Padmasana

Seated, lift each foot and cross onto each thigh. Try both sides.

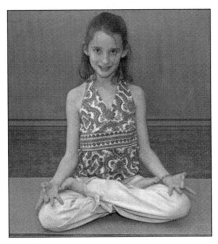

Lotus Pose

Benefits

Helps with relaxation and calms the mind. Opens the hips.

What it looks like

Lotus, any flower, a fairy, a meditating Genie.

MOUNTAIN POSE
Tadasana

Stand with feet fist–width apart. Weight evenly distributed through all four corners of the feet. Muscles of the ankles, calves, knees and thighs engaged and hugging the bones. Inner thighs are back, tailbone tucked. Shoulders are on the back, hands pointed down. Feel the energy from the earth and feet drawing up into the core and extending out through the hands and head and feet.

Benefits

Naturally aligns the entire body. Spinal alignment. Teaches proper standing. Develops concentration. Makes back strong. Relaxing.

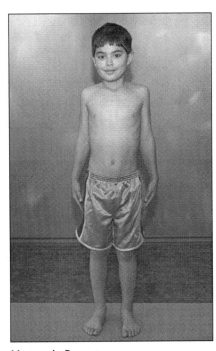

Mountain Pose

What it looks like

A steady mountain, a torpedo.

ONE LEG HEAD TO KNEE POSE
Janu Shirsasana

Begin sitting and bring one bent knee in and extend other leg out. Draw in with the inner thighs and extend out through the feet. Extend forward and bring chest to thigh.

Benefits

Stretches and strengthens hamstrings. Tones kidneys and liver. Heart is at rest.

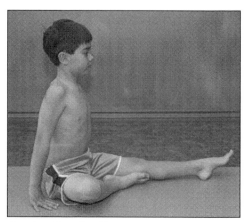

One Leg Head to Knee Pose

What it looks like

Branches, an arrow.

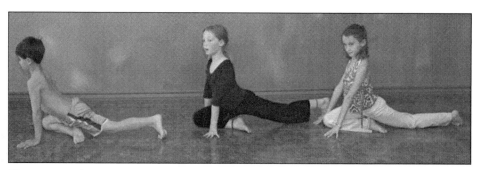

Pigeon Pose

PIGEON POSE
Eka Pada Rajakapotasana prep

Begin in **table position**. Bring one knee forward and extend back leg out, activate back leg. Extend up. Bow forward. Switch sides.

Benefits

Opens the hips. Stretches the legs. Opens the heart.

What it looks like

Someone crawling on the ground, a seal, a pigeon, ice skating.

RABBIT POSE

Begin in **table position**. Place hands on ankles, then arch the back and tuck head under. Place gentle weight on head.

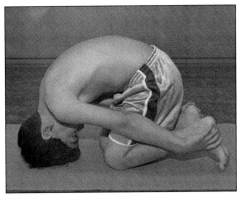

Rabbit Pose

Benefits

Stretches the back, arms and neck.

What it looks like

A rabbit, a butter ball, a bomb, a seed.

RAINBOW POSE
Urdva Dhanurasana

Place hands behind shoulders before pressing up into **bridge pose**. Come up onto head, draw shoulders on to back, curl under, then press up with hands into full pose.

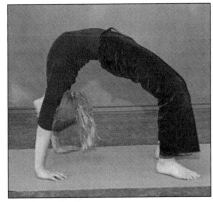

Rainbow Pose

Benefits

Good for rounded shoulders and back. Aids respiration. Improves energy. Opens heart. Strengthens arms, shoulders and wrists. Makes back flexible.

What it looks like

A wheel, a rainbow, a tunnel, a magic portal through an invisible door in the wall.

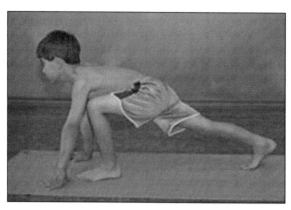
Runner's Lunge

RUNNER'S LUNGE

Begin in **table position** or **downward dog.** and lunge right foot forward with knee at a right angle above the ankle. Bring shoulders on the back and extend out through back foot.

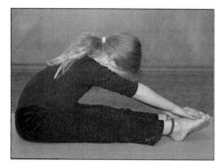
Seated Forward Bend

SEATED FORWARD BEND
Paschimotanasana

Sit on floor with legs extended. Activate legs and inner thighs. Bow forward and touch toes.

Benefits

Tones the abdominal organs, kidneys and is good for the spine. Lengthens hamstrings.

What it looks like

A flower getting ready to bloom, a shy animal.

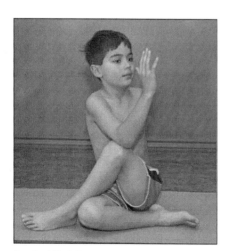
Seated Twist

SEATED TWIST
Ardha Matsydendrasana I

Begin seated with legs extended. Bend left knee and place foot over the opposite leg. Bring opposite foot in toward buttocks. Cross right elbow to left knee and leverage back. Reverse.

Benefits

Stretches neck muscles. Tones the internal organs. Good for the spine and shoulders. Releases toxins.

What it looks like

A pretzel, a mixed–up professor, looking this way and that way.

SIDE ANGLE POSE
Parsvakonasana

Begin with legs wide apart on the mat. Turn left foot in 60 degrees, and extend right foot out straight. Bend right knee to about a 90 degree angle, bring arm and elbow either down to the right knee or down to the outside of the right ankle. Extend left arm up over head, pinky pointing down. Reverse.

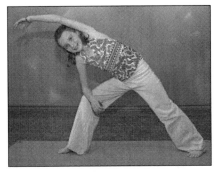

Side Angle Pose

Benefits

Builds stamina. Good for toning ankles, knees and thighs. Develops the chest and opens the shoulders.

What it looks like

Traveling up and down hills, going places, a leaning tree.

SPLITS
Hanumanasana

Begin in **runner's lunge**. Slowly walk front leg out in front, maintaining muscular energy.

Benefits

Tones leg muscles. Good for sciatica.

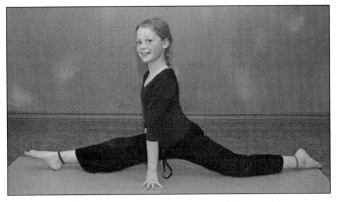

Splits

What it looks like

A cheerleader, a monkey, a road runner, a ballerina.

TABLE POSITION

Begin on hands and knees, toes untucked, fingers spread wide, wrist joints straight across. Back with natural curve.

TREE POSE
Vrksasana

Begin in **mountain pose**. Put weight onto left leg and then lift right foot to the left thigh, toes pointing downwards. Balancing, lift arms up over head, palms together. Flower the tree by opening the hands and bring arms down to the sides again. Switch sides.

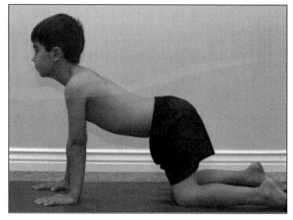

Table Position

Benefits

Develops balance and concentration, and tones the leg muscles.

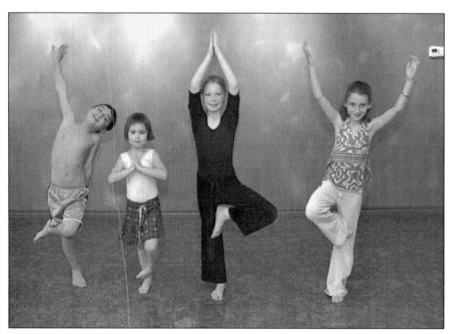

Tree Pose

What it looks like

A tree, a rocket ship.

TRIANGLE POSE
Trikonasana

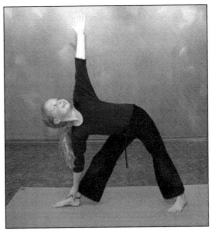

Spread legs wide on the mat, left foot turned in at 60 degrees and right foot pointing straight out. Inhale arms up to shoulder height. Bring muscular energy to the legs and arms, then extend trunk over to the right leg and bring the right hand toward the right shin, ankle or mat. Left arm extends straight up. Look at the fingertips. Switch sides.

Triangle Pose

Benefits

Strengthens leg muscles and ankles. Builds and opens the chest.

What it looks like

Traveling places, a triangle, a magic wand.

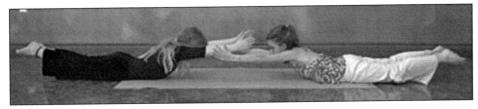

Upward Boat

UPWARD BOAT
Urdva Navasana

Lying on stomach with both arms extended out front, arch back and lift off arms and legs from ground. Extend out through hands and feet.

Benefits

Good for the back. Tones the abdominal organs.

What it looks like

A magic carpet, a flying fish, a boat, Superman, Superwoman.

WARRIOR I
Virabhadrasana I

Spread legs wide. Turn left foot in 60 degrees and right foot out 90 degrees. Turn hips. Bend left knee to a 90 degree angle, extend arms up over head. Reverse sides.

Benefits

Opens up and strengthens shoulders, back and neck. Develops good breathing in the chest. Builds stamina, strengthens legs, ankles and knees. Stretches thighs.

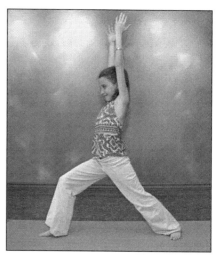

Warrior I

What it looks like

Any major or minor character, proud warrior, victorious runner.

WARRIOR II
Virabhadrasana II

Spread legs wide. Turn left foot in 60 degrees and right foot out 90 degrees. Bend right knee toward a 90 degree angle, extend right arms out in front and left arm behind. Look toward right fingertips. Reverse sides.

Benefits

Opens up and strengthens shoulders, back and neck. Develops good breathing in the chest. Builds stamina, strengthens legs, ankles and knees.

What it looks like

Any major or minor character, proud warrior, Egyptian dancer.

WARRIOR III
Virabhadrasana III

Begin in **Warrior I** position. Take a small step forward with back right foot. Balance on left foot. Interlace hands together, index fingers and thumbs together and extend arms and hands out in front. Lift and extend right leg straight out behind. Arms can also be at the side. Reverse sides.

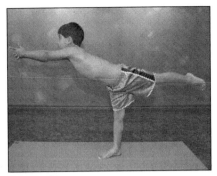

Warrior III

Benefits

Opens up and strengthens shoulders, back and neck. Develops good breathing in the chest. Builds stamina and balance, strengthens legs, ankles and knees.

What it looks like

Any major or minor character, an arrow, an airplane, a flying warrior.

WIDE ANGLE POSE
Upavistha Konasana

Sitting on floor with legs straight in front, open legs to the side, toes pointing up if possible, and bow forward.

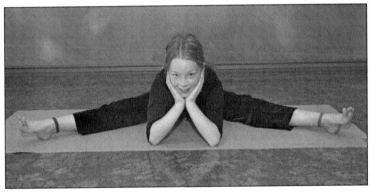

Wide Angle Pose

Benefits

Stretches the hamstrings and legs.

What it looks like

A lazy princess, a doorway to another world.

MORE FUN WITH STORY AND YOGA

Finding and Using Stories to Add Asanas To

Read lots of juvenile fiction and books about folktales, myths and fairy tales. They are in the juvenile library under 398.2. If you use a picture book, you can show the book and pictures after creating the story with yoga.

Look for stories that illustrate a theme or have concrete images or actions to readily draw upon to illustrate known yoga postures. If you find a story that has a moon, a tree, a dog, etc., that's great, but it's not always necessary. The important thing is to relate the story or character through the symbol of a physical posture.

For example, for the *Diamonds, Rubies and Pearls* story a pose such as feather dancer, *natarajasana,* or camel pose, *ustrasana,* sort of makes the shape of a diamond or a pearl. Really, your imagination is the limit. You will be surprised what kinds of images kids attach to postures. Downward dogs become tents and mountains. Upward boats become seals, magic carpets, boomerangs, etc.

Standing poses are a central part of yoga practice. All of the warrior poses, *virabhradrasana I, II, III,* can easily be introduced at the beginning because the story always has a central character and hero. It can also be used whenever another central character appears.

Use triangle pose, *trikonasana,* or side angle pose, *parshvakonasana,* to illustrate movement or traveling. But you can do anything you want! During a six– or eight–week program, encourage children to practice by making up their own stories with asanas at home. They can demonstrate it for the whole class. You will be amazed at their creativity.

Remember to ask them:

Who is the main character, hero or heroine?

What do they want?

What kinds of obstacles are in the way?

What happens next?

What happens at the end to solve the problem?

For older children, add extra forward bends, downward dogs, forward lunges, etc. to move into other poses. With preschool children, stick with the basic poses and make it as simple as possible.

Making Up Stories With Asanas

Another fun way to combine story with yoga is to have children make up stories while doing the yoga practice. Asking the basic story questions from above, have children create the story with poses.

"Who is the story about?"

"A king, a princess, etc." Add a pose. Chair pose once became a princess with a fluffy dress.

"What are they doing? What do they want?"

"She's sad and tired,"

"Why?"

"She needs to get out of the house because her father, the king, is a pain."

Traveling poses. Triangle, side angle pose, etc. Warrior poses for the king.

"Then what happened?"

"She saw a snake and a crow." Snake and crow (*bakasana*) poses (not in book).

"Then what happened?"

"They told the king about a treasure."

"What's in the way of him finding the treasure?"

"A terrible dragon." Lion's pose, or make a dragon face.

"Then what happened?"

"He threw magic dust that the crow gave him onto the dragon and the dragon became his friend and showed him where the treasure was, through a magic door." Treasure, bound angle pose, then, shoulder stand with legs opening became the magic door.

"What was in the treasure chest?" Any variety of answers!

"How does the story end?"

"She's rich and doesn't have to go back to her dad. She starts her own ice cream parlor with the dragon." Ending with any pose, bringing hands back to heart space, *anjali mudra*.

What's That Pose?

This is a great way to introduce more poses and also to get kids' imaginations going.

Strike a pose and have kids use their imaginations about what the pose could be: people, objects, places, etc. Make up a story with the poses.

Warmup Stories

Show two or three different poses suitable for warmups. Choose a child to make up a story with those poses and have the child teach the class a warmup with it.

Make up your own chants, warmups and songs!

Add On

Have children add on and call out poses as you tell a story.

Name that Pose

Have children name the poses in Spanish or Sanskrit.

Fairy Tale *Shavasana* – upper elementary

During a series of *shavasana*, children create a fairy tale. After the story is complete the children add poses to the story and teach the story and yoga to the class.

After each *shavasana* segment have children discuss their segments of the story. Encourage children to watch their dreams at night and write them down during this exercise.

1) You are in your safe place. Imagine your safe place. (see Safe Place exercise) Something is wrong in the surrounding town where you live. Someone has taken something away and it has affected the town and its people. What is it that is taken away? Who took it away and why? What effect does it have on the people? On you?

2) Somebody comes and tells you that you must go on a journey and recover that which has been taken away. Who is that person? Where do you have to go? You set out on a path.

What is that path? Where are you going?

3) You meet an animal. What kind of an animal is it? The animal leads you to a special cave. You go into the cave and see diamonds on the ground, leading you into the cave. You sit down when the diamonds end. Something happens in the cave. What is it? Is there a person? An event? When the event or person is finished, there are three magic objects left for you to keep. What are the magic objects?

4) You continue on your journey with your animal friend to recover that which was taken. However, something difficult is in your way and you cannot continue. What is in your way? Is it a flaming lake? A brick wall 100 miles wide and 100 miles tall? Is it 10,000 hungry monkeys attacking you? Use one of your magic objects to solve the problem. You continue on your journey, and again there is an obstacle. What is it? Use the second magic object to solve the problem and continue on your journey. A third problem comes up. What is it? Use the third magic object to solve the problem and continue on your way.

5) Your special animal friend cannot go with you any farther. Where is it going? Why can't it go any farther? But the animal gives you a powerful gift. It can make you invisible, super strong, psychic, etc. What is the magic, powerful gift the animal gives you?

6) Continue on your journey to the place where you need to recover that which has been taken. You must recover it. Who do you encounter and what do you do to get the item back?

7) You return home to restore the town with that which had been taken. How does it feel to have it restored? How does the town react? What is different?

8) You go to a special place. What and where is that place? You meet somebody there. Who is it? You plan on staying there for a while to learn something. How long do you stay? What do you learn? What do you do with what you learned and the person you are with?

Have children write and tell their stories, add yoga poses, then teach the class the story and yoga.

Using Stories to Teach Themes in Yoga

Stories can also be used in yoga classes not only to be acted out as poses, but also to enrich the practice itself. To this end, they can be used to set the theme.

Bring up the theme throughout the class at different times for children to contemplate. Ask children periodically about how and what they feel.

For example, the story *Blind Men and the Elephant* in Heather Forest's *Wisdom Tales From Around the World* can be used to teach about differences in perceptions and opinions, as well as relying on inner instincts. During poses have a child breathe in the words, "I trust my inner wisdom. I am confident in myself." Children can talk about a time when their opinion was different from another's. How did they solve the argument?

Use the blindfold game for children to search out people and demonstrate inner reliance. Afterward ask them how they felt.

For a theme about letting go, surrendering and trusting: *The Story of the Sand* From *Tales of the Dervishes,* by Idries Shah, is about letting go, not being afraid and trusting in the higher self. Children can contemplate letting go during yoga, and not try to be perfect. How can you let go during your daily life? Are you under pressure to perform or compete? Use affirmations to say, "I find peace. I let go. I am OK."

Nasrudin is the Sufi trickster and fool. His stories are funny and kids love them. A theme can be that we do yoga to have fun. We don't have to be perfect or hard on ourselves if we fall down during yoga, because that's part of the fun! We do our own yoga and honor ourselves.

To emphasize truth (*satya*), honesty and self-confidence, Demi's *The Empty Pot* is a wonderful story.

For a theme about non–judgment *The Cherry Blossom* story in *Zen Stories for all Ages* by Martin Rafe is useful. We learn not to judge ourselves when difficult things happen to others or us, and not to judge ourselves when doing yoga. We treat others and ourselves with loving kindness and compassion. During the class if a child falls over and does something silly, remind them of the story and how it relates to the present moment. We never know how things will turn out!

After class, gather children around for more related stories and storytelling to fill time or for an extended class. Include wisdom stories of many faiths to compare and contrast ideas, as well as to develop children's tolerance toward others. Children can draw pictures about the stories they heard or make up more stories.

Additional Tips and Ideas for Teaching Yoga

After a cycle of the stories given in this book it's fine to repeat them. Children love to hear the same stories over and over again. It is through repetition that children are able to internalize the story, its structure and its meaning. Children will often be excited to hear the story again and say, "Oh, that's my favorite!" Through repitition the child can retell the story.

As children progress in yoga, if you have more time or if you are working with older children, introduce more yoga poses. Remember, children are very flexible and as they continue strengthening their bodies with yoga, they can do advanced poses.

Introduce one or two new poses in each class. Ask children what kinds of people, objects or animals the pose reminds them of. Have them do the poses as "home fun" to practice.

Take time to adjust children in the poses, emphasizing correct alignment with feet, knees and ankles, etc.

Add variations to the sun salutations, such as an additional warrior or twist.

Have children strike their favorite yoga pose.

Have them choose a pose from the story and act it out.

Ask them to keep a dream journal. What kinds of dreams are coming up? Make up stories using their dreams!

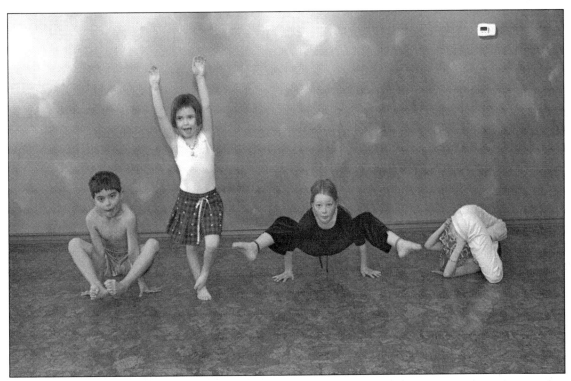

Kids striking their favorite yoga pose.

GAMES

Tummy Spin

On a smooth floor, swing both legs over to right. Then use tummy muscles to pull and swing both legs to the left to build momentum. Repeat a few times until enough momentum is built up to use tummy muscles to pull legs into chest and spin.

Tummy Game

Have children place their head onto one another's belly, creating a crooked line. Have all the children laugh. The feel of the heads on the tummies and tummies on the heads will entertain the kids and they will laugh more, causing a chain reaction. We are all connected!

Atom Game

Start children milling around by themselves in different directions. Call out a number between one and four (according to the size of the group.) A group must form with that number of children. Continue calling out different numbers and having them mill around. This even works with small groups of about five. Young ones just love to count and get together rather than worry about exact numbers.

Variation: have kids connect at elbows, knees, feet, etc.

Ball Game and Shanti Chant

Shanti means peace.

Shanti, Shanti in me and you.
Peace, peace in all we do.

Throw a ball to a child. Have her tell something good about herself. Something she likes to do, a talent, a personality trait. Little kids can talk about things they like to do or a favorite toy. Have her pass the ball to another child and repeat.

Variation: Call out parts of the body that the child must use, elbow, chin, knee, bottom, etc. in order to send the ball over to the next child.

Balance Game

Play music and have children dance around. Stop music. Children must stop in tracks and balance on one foot and whatever position they are in.

Blindfold Game

Blindfold a child and have them search for friends in a circle and try and guess whom they touch. Older children can call to the younger ones to aid their search. This game develops inner sensory awareness and is great to use with the story *The Blind Men and the Elephant.*

Balloon Game

Send a blown up balloon around the room with children hitting it using one part of their body only, such as head, elbows, knee or chin.

Hula Hoop Game

Have children hold hands in a circle. Children have to pass their body through the hula–hoop without letting go of each other's hands. The hula–hoop gets passed on down the line.

For advanced or older children, try a thick rope or string.

Races

Crab race. Penguin race — walking on knees, holding onto ankles. Monkey race — scuttle across floor like a monkey. Wheelbarrow race.

Dance

Put on fun music and dance around the room! Children love to express their bodies.

Shadow Dancing

Put on interesting music, such as Japanese flute music. In a darkened room, shine a flashlight against the wall. Have children make up a story with the movement of their body and the shadows they create.

Eye Gazing

Pair children up. Have them look into each other's eyes. They will laugh, but ask them to try and get beyond laughing. Have them look deeply into the other's eyes and see if they can see themselves in the eyes of the other. Then have one child put hand on shoulders so he can feel a connection to the other child. Then have him pull their ears gently. Switch. Have them talk about how this felt.

Memory Game

Have child pick a partner and look at them very closely, noting every detail about what they are wearing, eye color, etc. Have the child then close their eyes and recall it back to the partner. Switch.

Hand and Mantra Game

Using classic hand game, sing mantras to the tune of *row, row, row your boat*, or *here we go around the mulberry bush*. Use mantras such as *Om Namashivaya*. You can use any religious or non–religious mantra of your choice.

Two children face each other. One child can hold still while the other claps, or both children can move their hands simultaneously. Clap hands together. Right hand crosses over to facing child's right hand. Clap hands together again. Left hand crosses over to facing child's left hand. Clap hands together twice, clap back of hands against facing child's back of hands, flip hands over and clap palms of both hands against facing child's hands. Repeat.

Singing Mantras

Sing mantras out loud, repeating over and over.

Chant *Hare Krsna, Hare Krsna, Krsna Krsna, Hare Hare, Hare Rama, Hare Rama, Rama Rama, Hare Hare* to simple nursery rhyme tunes such as *row, row, row your boat*. You can use any religious or non–religious mantra of your choice.

Or

Jesus loves me this I know, for the Bible tells me so.
Yes, Jesus loves me. Yes, Jesus loves me.

MEDITATION

Meditation is the last limb of yoga before *samadhi*, or self–realization. After developing children's character, bodies, breath and developing their concentration, they move closer to the goal of yoga, union with the divine. That self–awareness that yes, I am divine here on this earth in this body.

I teach children that with yoga and meditation we find that center within us. That we are like a wheel, with a center. We move from the center and our work becomes effortless and beautiful. There is no stress, fear or doubt. Our desires, or *kama*, can be fulfilled. The result is that whatever we set our minds to do, be it school work, athletics, art, music or any other desire, it will be done with excellence and joy.

Inside Awareness Chant

Inside, inside with my third eye I see myself clearly
Outside, outside eyes open wide I send love to all dearly
Om Amen

Hand Watching Meditation

Begin in prayer position, *anjali mudra*, hands away from chest. Slowly let tips of fingers collapse on themselves inward. Curve down as backs of hands and fingers touch each other. Watch as hands become totally on backside and all the way down to the wrist.

Children are to do this as slowly as possible. Ask them to look at their hands. For preschool–aged children simply open and close hands like a flower beginning at fingers all the way down to the wrists.

Wave Breathing Meditation

With eyes closed imagine breathing in like a wave that is going out to sea. Breathing out, be like the wave, breathing all the way to the shore. Bring breath back in and make for a strong and beautiful wave and then out again to caress the shore. Repeat several times.

Wave Meditation

Have children open their eyes. Have them look to their right and look at everything around them, all the while being aware of the breath moving in and out. Call out in, out, like a wave, as they just look for a few minutes. Remind them to bring their attention back to the breath and to looking at the objects in the room if they are thinking about school or toys or something else rather than the real world in front of them.

Counting Meditation

Have children count using the breath. Inhale one, exhale two, inhale three, exhale four and so on. If they forget to count, have them start over with one. For preschool children, count inhale one, exhale two, inhale one, exhale two.

Expanding Meditation

Have children sit comfortably. Tell them to imagine that they are surrounded by beautiful white light. The light is so peaceful and safe and happy and loving. Every time they inhale, the white light fills them up. Every time they exhale the white light expands out farther. It expands to reach the other children. When they inhale, all that love and light comes back to them. Imagine the white light is touching and holding them, peaceful, loving and kind. Exhaling, it continues to expand to the room, then outside, to the street, to the whole city, then the whole state and the country, then the world, then the universe, farther and farther out to other galaxies. Then bring it back to the heart. Sit in silence.

Walking Meditation

Begin with the left hand in a fist, resting with the right hand around it. Looking down, have children slowly walk around the room in a circle for three minutes. Ask them to exaggerate the slowness of their movements, of the heels hitting the floor and then the ball of the foot stepping, moving to the toes, pressing off with the back big toe, picking up the foot to step and so on. Have them be very quiet and as slow as possible in walking. If they bunch up, tell them it's OK to walk to the side of another child.

Tell them that this is their own yoga. Remind them to breathe. You can see the children whose minds are wandering off into the clouds. Remind them to take their brilliant minds and put them into their bodies and the breath. Remind them to look at their feet and feel their body and breath.

Tell them that yoga and meditation is not just quiet time or just on the yoga mat. It is always! When they are in school, brushing their teeth, doing homework, being with family, riding in the car. It's an awareness of themselves and the present moment and their wonderful life. It's a wake–up call! In the moment! I'm breathing! When I'm breathing, I'm alive! It's great to be alive! It's great to be me!

Variation for preschoolers and up: Have children walk slowly, talk to them about moving slowly. Remind them to breathe. Ask them to look at their own feet, rather than a neighbor's. Then ring a bell and have children run around fast! If space is an issue, have them jump in place. Then ring the bell again, have them go slowly. Ring again. Fast! And so on.

Arm Moving Meditation

Children are standing with arms straight in front of them. Have them move the arms all the way over to their right in a gentle twist. Tell them that there is a beautiful, soft velvet curtain and they are going to touch that curtain and really feel it. Then, as slowly as they possibly can, keeping the arms and hands lifted, move the arms and hands back to center. Then children continue over to their left side, again, emphasizing a slow, continuous movement. Remind the children to breathe. Remind them to feel the curtain and to move very slowly.

Candle Meditation

Light a small candle in the room. Have children gaze and focus on it. Remind them to breathe.

For older children, ask them to contemplate: What is the candle made of? Where is the flame coming from? The candle is made of wax. Where does the wax come from? Bees. What do bees do? How do they make the wax? Continue with the wick, etc. How does the wick get to be in the candle? Always bring the mind back to the candle.

Bell Meditation

Appoint one child to ring the bell. You can use the bell ringer as a reward for children who concentrate and participate without disruption. The child must be patient to wait until the sound of the bell has faded completely before ringing the bell again. Instruct other children to listen completely and entirely to the bell sound.

Listening Meditation

Have children sit still, hands on lap and eyes closed. Have children listen attentively for one minute to all the sounds around them. After one minute have them share what they heard.

Hand Meditation and Song – see appendix for words and music

Right hand: Inhale, then bring thumb to index finger and exhale. Inhale, separate fingers again. Exhale, bring thumb to middle finger. Inhale, separate fingers. Exhale, bring thumb to ring finger. Inhale, separate fingers. Exhale thumb to pinky.

Inhale, then exhale and rest hand in lap and switch to other hand.

Preschool children may not be able to do finger touching and singing at the same time. They can choose to sing or open and close their hands.

Awareness Meditation

Have children in sitting position, crisscross applesauce. With eyes closed and hands on the lap, tell children to be aware of and feel the air coming in and out of their nostrils. Have them feel their bottoms on the earth, the air on their skin, the feeling of their clothes on their skin, their hands on the lap. Have them be aware of their head, eyes, nose, mouth.

Loving Kindness Meditation

Children can have their eyes open or closed. Repeat out loud.

May I be happy. May I be at Peace. May I be well. May I dwell in my heart. May my heart flower.

May you be happy. May you be at Peace. May you be well. May you dwell in your heart. May your heart flower.

May we be happy. May we be at Peace. May we be well. May we dwell in our hearts. May our hearts flower.

CREATIVE RELAXATION FOR CHILDREN

Relaxation, or *shavasana*, can be one of the most important aspects of yoga for children — especially children today, bombarded as they are, day in and day out, by the sound and imagery of advertising.

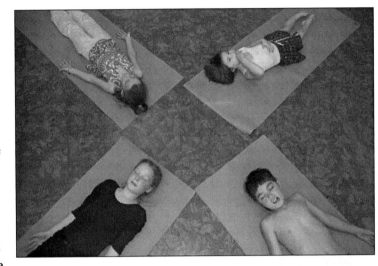

Additionally, *shavasana* may be the only quiet relaxation time children get all day.

Have children lie on their backs, arms away from their sides a bit, palms facing up. Legs should be slightly apart. Eye bags help eliminate distractions. Also a blanket may cover them to keep them warm. Many children will be able to lie still, and others will wiggle. Over time most children are able to get into the routine of relaxation.

Have children start by focusing on their breathing. Use a soft, soothing, slow voice and emphasize the in and out of the breath. For older children, instruct them to explore the gaps in the breath: The silence, emptiness and peacefulness.

Explain that our bodies are like batteries. When we rest, we are recharging our bodies with energy so that we can go out into the world and do more wonderful things.

Instruct them that if the mind wanders, see if they can catch it and label it as "thinking" and bring it back to the breath. Tell them to begin again and that it's OK if the mind wanders. Also have them try and look for the gap that is between the thoughts. Have them try and witness the space.

Most of all emphasize the breath moving in and out, and that at each exhalation the body sinks into the earth and relaxes. It lets go. There are no worries, nothing to do, nothing to achieve, nowhere to go. Use the breath of in and out, letting go and so forth throughout all these meditations. Always remind the children to come back to their bodies, back to their breath.

Children who are especially wiggly can be urged to put their hands on their stomach and/or heart and feel the breath. I remind kids that if they are wiggling around, their monkey is running wild. Kids also can be rewarded for being still by having the honor of ringing the bell when it's time to get up.

The Floppy Test

After children have taken a position lying down, say you are going to do the "Floppy Test" to see who is really relaxed. Choose a child and pick up his arm and flop it around to see if he is really relaxed. If there is tension or muscular energy, tell him to "Get floppy! Let go!" If the child is relaxed say, "Now here's a relaxed and floppy yogi!" Continue with a few other children.

For Preschool Children and Up

Peace and Joy Breath

1) While in *shavasana*, breathe in "yes," to my life. Breathe out "love" or "peace."

2) Breathe in "happy." Exhale "joy."

Relax

Have children clench fist of their right arm. Super tight! Then let go. Let it all relax. Have them clench their whole arm and fist, then let go.

Continue going through all the parts of the body, chest, to the legs, then the other leg, foot, other arm and hand, then the head, each time clenching each part super tight with all their might, then letting go. Finally have them clench the whole body, super tight! Then let go. Relax. Sink into the earth.

Feather

There is a beautiful bird sitting on a branch. The bird opens its colorful wings and flies upward, floating easy in the sky, free, happy. A feather comes loose. You are that feather. Be the feather, as it slowly, slowly, rocks back and forth in the air, floating downward toward the earth. Back and forth you go, floating, floating. Then you land on the earth, light, happy, relaxed.

Cloud

Imagine that you are resting on a cloud. The cloud is so fluffy and soft, so puffy and light. Feel that cloud under you. It's like a little bed. The cloud is just floating in the sky, sailing along. There are no worries, nothing to do. It gently floats through the sky with you on it.

Big Sky

You are lying in a beautiful meadow with lovely flowers all around you. You look up into the sky and see little birds singing and flying by. The sky is so big and beautiful blue. There are no clouds at all. But there is a little black dot up there in that big sky. Just look at that black dot in the big, blue sky.

Sand

Imagine that you are lying on the beach. The beautiful sky and sun are above you. Imagine that sand is filling up your toes and feet. Your toes and feet get so heavy, filled with this sand. They are so heavy they can't move. They are relaxed and sink into the earth. Then the sand moves up your calves and fills them up. They are heavy and sink into the earth. You feel so heavy and relaxed. You let go. Breathing in and out. Then the sand moves up to your knees, to your thighs and fills them up with sand. You are so heavy with sand that you can't move your legs. Then the sand moves up to your chest and all the way up to your neck. Sand is filling you up. You sink into the earth. Relaxed, peaceful. Then the sand moves into your arms, all the way down to your fingers. You are so relaxed and heavy. You let go and sink into the earth. The sand comes up to your face, relaxes your mouth, your eyes, your checks, your scalp. They all fill up with sand and sink into the earth. You relax and are so heavy. Your whole body sinks into the earth. You feel calm and peaceful. Breathing in and breathing out.

Sunshine

Imagine that you are lying on the beach. Breathe into your heart and imagine that inside your heart is a beautiful sun. The sun is so warm and it warms up your whole body. Then exhale and the sun comes up above you. The sun shines down on you and you feel its wonderful, golden warmth. The sun's rays touch your toes and feet, and they soak up the sun's light and feel so heavy and warm, they sink into the sand. Down, down, into the earth you go. Happy, safe, peaceful, relaxed.

The sun moves up your calves, your legs, and they soak up the golden sun, and they are heavy and sink into the earth. The sun moves up your hips, stomach, chest, and they just soak up the sun and feel so warm and heavy. They sink into the earth. The sun moves up to your neck, down your arms, into your elbows and fingers. They are heavy, filled with golden light, warmth and happiness. You sink into the earth. You let go. The sun goes all the way up to your head, relaxes your lips, jaw, cheeks, eyes, forehead, scalp. It feels so warm, golden, happy. You sink into the earth. Your whole body is filled with the beautiful, radiant, golden light of the sun. You breathe in the sun back into your heart. And you are relaxed, golden, heavy, happy.

Imagine somebody that you love. Somebody who makes you very happy. Smile at them. Then imagine somebody that you don't like, somebody who gives you trouble. Smile at them. Then see yourself. Smile at yourself. Then see something about yourself that you don't like, something you don't feel good about. Smile at this thing. Smile at yourself. Then take the hand of the person you love very much, and the person who gives you trouble and all three of you go to the place you want to go most in the world. Where is it? What do you do? What things are happening? What sights, sounds and smells?

Still Pond

Imagine a pond of cool water. Throw a stone in it. See the stone sink to the bottom of the pond. Feel your body, heavy as the stone, sinking, down, down, down. Relaxed. Happy. Peaceful. See the ripples on the pond. Watch them go to the shore. Then see all the ripples disappear, one by one. Until there are no more ripples. Just see the clear, motionless pond. See it all in your mind's eyes.

Flower Heart

Imagine a flower in your heart. What kind of a flower is it? See its color, beauty and smell. Now see that it is in a tiny, beautiful bud. With every breath you take imagine that the flower is opening petal by petal. Every breath you take, you feel full, held and secure. Every exhalation let go and feel your body drop down into the earth as if the flower had roots that are reaching deep down into the earth. Drop like a stone thrown into a pond. Down, down it goes. Then breathe in again into the heart, open the petals a little bit more, and again, exhaling the roots down deeper into the earth. Repeat until the petals are all the way open and the flower is blooming. Look inside the flower. What do you see? What's there in the middle of the flower? Then see yourself in that flower. Happy, smiling, safe, secure.

Dreaming

Breathing in and out. Breathe in calm. Breathe out ease. Breathe in happy. Breathe out love.

Breathe in peace. Breathe out joy.

See yourself doing something that you've always wanted to do. Something that you're good at. Or something that you want to become when you are older. What is it? It could be something you are about to do in the future, or something that's going to happen. What dream of yourself are you bringing into the world? What is your passion? See yourself participating, doing it masterfully. Feel how happy you are doing that which you love to do and doing it beautifully.

Expanding

Close your eyes. Look down with your inner eye to the heart. Feel the breath move in and out. Then see yourself in your heart and say to yourself: "I love myself. I trust myself. I lovingly give, and I lovingly receive back." Then see somebody that you love. Send your love to them. Feel them sending love back to you. See somebody you don't like. Send them love. Feel them give you love back. Then breathe in feeling love, then breathe out, and send the love into the room, beyond your body. To all the people around you. Breathe in and feel them giving you love back. That love you receive is just as big as the love that you sent out. On the out breath, expand outward to the whole school; on the in breath feel the love coming back to you, the love of the whole school coming into you. Say to yourself, "I am loved." Exhale again and expand outward toward the whole city, the whole state, the country, the earth, and the whole universe into infinity. When you breathe in, you receive infinity back to yourself in love. You are infinity. Say to yourself: "I am loved. I am love. I am peace. I am peace."

For Elementary

Diamond Cave

Imagine that you are barefoot walking through the woods. Feel the soft, green forest floor beneath your feet. Look up and see the tops of the trees and the sun streaming through them. You notice an animal. What kind of an animal is it? Watch it walk away and show you down a little path. You feel safe and happy, and follow the animal along the path. You go to a cave. The cave is lit with little diamonds along the way. Follow the animal into the cave, feeling safe and happy as you follow the diamonds lighting the way. The diamonds stop and you find yourself in the middle of the cave. Then a little window opens up from above and beautiful light pours down on you. It bathes you in love, safety and happiness. Make a wish. Anything that you want. Anything that you most want in the world or want to do. Say thank you, and then set it free, knowing that your wish has been heard. Then relax. Rest. Come out of the cave, go back down the path. Now lie down in a beautiful meadow and rest.

Sunshine and Sunflowers

Imagine planting a seed at the bottom of your spine. Water the seed with your breath. Each time you inhale the plant begins to grow. Now imagine the seed right below your stomach. It rests there for a moment and then begins to grow again upward. With every breath, it moves into your tummy, then into your heart, then up to your throat, then in the middle of your forehead. Now imagine a rolling field blooming with yellow sunflowers. You are the sunflower, gazing tall at the sky and earth. Now imagine taking a crown full of sunflowers and placing it on your head. In the crown imagine unfolding the sunflowers petal by petal and showering your body with golden light.

Sailing Away

Get in a little boat. Lie on your back. Feel the water rock you back and forth, back and forth, as if you were in your mother or father's arms rocking. Feel so peaceful, safe, relaxed. Breathing in and out. The sailboat gently rocks in the lake, floating, happy. It comes to a little island. You get up and look around. What is your island? What do you see? Somebody is there to greet you. They take you somewhere. Where is it? A city, a castle? A garden, a jungle? What do you see and visit? Who is there? Be there for a while. Explore this place for a while But then it's time to say good–bye. The greeter gives you a gift. What is it? What are you supposed to do with it? Thank them for the gift. Get in your boat, sail back home. Rocking back and forth. Slowly, slowly. Relax. Let go.

Body Points

Starting at the top of the head breathe in. Exhale down to the right leg. Inhale back to the head, exhale to the left leg. Inhale to the head, exhale to the tailbone. Inhale to the head, exhale to the stomach. Inhale to the head, exhale to the heart. Inhale to the head, exhale to the right hand. Inhale to the head, exhale to the left hand. Inhale to the head, exhale to the neck. Inhale to the head, exhale to the forehead. Inhale and exhale to the top of the head. Then release. Bring focus back to the heart.

Ending Shavasana

Give about 2–5 minutes for quiet time and then sing the breathing song quietly to them. Ring the bell and tell children to start wiggling their toes and hands and then to inhale and stretch arms over head. Bring knees to chin and give self a hug, then roll over on right side and rest. Then use arms to pull up to sitting.

After *shavasana* have children talk about their experiences and tell stories about what they did, where they went and how they felt. Encourage them to give details and bring out more parts of the story by asking, what happened next?

Encourage them to write stories, write down dreams, paint pictures, draw, sculpt, whatever they wish to express their experiences while in *shavasana*.

ENDINGS

Ending Class

Ask a few children to tell the main story back to you. One person can do the beginning, the others the middle and the end. Coach them along with details or story elements if you need to.

After each child tells his part, ask him to show the class a pose that he remembers from that part of the story. Encourage children to practice those poses at home.

Have a child who has behaved well and participated, or the most improved, have the honor of ringing the bell, or saying goodbye to the puppet or object. They can put it away in its special box if there is one.

Heaven and Earth

Children in cross legged position to begin. Thumbs and index fingers together to form a triangle. Beginning at the base of the spine — "I am." Next, bringing hands into prayer position, *anjali mudra*, in front of heart — "I am love." Then, hands reach over the head, with thumbs and index fingers together again, palms facing away — "I am light." Bending at the elbow, right hand up, index finger and thumb together — "I am heaven." Left hand, index finger and thumb together, pointing down — "I am earth." Bring both hands up at sides, bending at the elbows. Make circles with hands and forearms — "I am creation." Reverse circle directions — "I am destruction." Reverse again — "I am creation." Arms crossing in front of body — "I am a child of God (light, love, etc.)." Release arms and reach into the sky. Bring arms back in cross in front of body. Remain in silence for a few seconds.

End with Namaste

The ritual of yoga is over, as all students bring hands into prayer position, *anjali mudra*, and bow out in namaste.

Thanks so much for reading the Storytime Yoga manual! Be sure to visit the Storytime Yoga web site and sign up for *The Lotus***, an E-zine filled with the latest news, stories and ideas to keep children healthy and happy! Sign up at www.StorytimeYoga.com and also receive the latest posts of new stories scripted with yoga!**

May you find joy, peace, happiness and fulfillment in sharing yoga and story with little ones!

OM SHANTI.

Sydney

RESOURCES

YOGA AND MEDITATION RESOURCES

Brunhoff, Laurent de. *Yoga for Elephants*. New York: Harry N. Abrams, 2002.

Chanchani, Rajiv, and Swati Chanchani. *Yoga for Children*. New Delhi: UBS Pub. Dist. Ltd., 1995.

Children of Yogaville. *Hatha Yoga for Kids, by Kids!* Buckingham: Integral Yoga, 1990.

Cohen, Kenneth K. *Imagine That! A Child's Guide to Yoga*. Buckingham: Integral Yoga, 1983.

Garth, Maureen. *Starbright, Meditations for Children*. Australia: Harper and Collins, 1994.

Iyengar, B.K.S. *Light on Yoga*. New York: Shocken Books, 1966.

Kaur Khalsa, Shakta. *Fly Like A Butterfly, Yoga for Children*. Portland: Rudra Press, 1998

Lark, Liz. *Yoga for Young People*. New York: Sterling Publishing, 2003.

Luby, Thia. *Children's Book of Yoga: Games & Exercises Mimic Plants & Animals & Objects*. Don Diego: Clear Light, 1998.

MacLean, Kerry Lee. *Peaceful Piggy Meditation*. Morton Grove: Albert Whitman, 2004.

Mipham, Sakyong. *Turning the Mind Into an Ally*. New York: Riverhead Books, 2003.

Radha, Swami Sivananda. *Hatha Yoga: The Hidden Language — Symbols, Secrets and Metaphor*. Spokane: Timeless Books, 1995.

Yoga Journal – www.yogajournal.com
Yoga International Magazine – www.yimag.com

Anusara Yoga – www.anusara.com
Radiant Yoga for Children – www.susankramer.com/yoga.html
YogaKids International – www.yogakids.com

www.braingym.com
www.storytimeyoga.com
www.mythicyoga.com

STORYTELLING RESOURCES

Bauer, Caroline Feller. *New Handbook for Storytellers*. Chicago: ALA, 1993.

Bayat, Mojdeh, and Jamnia Mohammad. *Tales from the Land of the Sufis*. Boston: Shambhala, 2001.

Bennett, William J. *The Children's Book of Virtues*. New York: Simon, 1995.

---. *The Moral Compass*. New York: Simon, 1995.

---. *The Book of Virtues*. New York: Simon, 1995.

Bhakta, Amal. *Mystical Stories from the Mahabharata: Twenty Timeless Lessons in Wisdom and Virtue*. Badger: Torchlight Publishing, 2000.

Cox, Allison M., and David H. Albert, eds. *The Healing Heart: Storytelling to Encourage Caring and Healthy Families.* Garviola Island, BC: New Society Publishers, 2003.

Conover, Sarah, Kindness. *A Treasury of Buddhist Widsom for Children and Parents.* Spokane: Eastern Washington UP, 2001.

Chodzin, Sherab, and Alexandra Koh. *The Wisdom of the Crows and other Buddhist Tales.* Bristol, UK: Barefoot Books, 1998.

Demi. *Buddha Stories.* New York: Henry Holt, 1997.

Dormer, Cindy. *Hold that Thought For Kids: Capturing Precious Memories Through Fun Questions, Images and Conversations.* Englewood: Brightside, 2004.

Edwards, Carolyn McVickar. *In the Light of the Moon: Thirteen Lunar Tales from Around the World Illuminating Life's Mysteries.* New York: Marlowe, 2003.

Forest, Heather. *Wisdom Tales from Around the World.* N.p.: August House, 1996.

Holt, David, and Bill Mooney. *Ready-to-Tell Tales: Surefire Stories from America's Favorite Storytellers.* N.p.: August House, 1994.

Lupton, Hugh. *Tales of Wisdom and Wonder.* Bristol, UK: Barefoot Books, 1998.

MacDonald, Margaret Read. *Peace Tales: World Folktales to Talk About.* Hamden: Linnet, 1992.

Maguire, Jack. *The Power of Personal Storytelling: Spinning Tales to Connect with Others.* New York: Putnam, 1998.

Millman, Lawrence. *A Kayak Full of Ghosts: Eskimo Folk Tales.* Northhampton: Interlink, 2004.

Martin, Rafe. *One Hand Clapping: Zen Stories for All Ages.* New York: Rizzoli, 1995.

McDermott, Gerald. Everything by this Caldecott-Winning Author.

Meade, Erica Helm. *The Moon in the Well: Wisdom Tales to Transform Your Life, Family, and Community.* Peru: Carus Publishing, 2001.

Mormon Church. *Family Home Evening Resource Book.* Salt Lake City: Mormon Church, 1983.

Murdoch, Maureen. *Spinning Inward: Using Guided Imagery with Children for Learning, Creativity and Relaxation.* Boston: Shambhala, 1997.

Otto, Gina. *Cassandra's Angel.* Denver: Gina's Ink, 2001.

Pearmain, Elisa Davy. *Doorways to the Soul: 52 Wisdom Tales from Around the World.* Cleveland: Pilgrim Press, 1998.

Pellowski, Anne. *The Storytelling Handbook.* New York: Simon, 1995.

Ragan, Kathleen. *Fearless Girls, Wise Women and Beloved Sisters: Heroines in Folktales from Around the World.* New York: Norton, 1998.

Roberts, Moss. *Chinese Fairy Tales and Fantasies.* New York: Pantheon, 1979.

Schwartz, Howard. *Elijah's Violin and Other Jewish Fairy Tales.* New York: Harper, 1983.

Shivkumar. *Stories From Panchatantra.* New Delhi: Children's Book Trust, 1994.

Shah, Idries, *Tales of the Dervishes.* New York: Penguin, 1993.

---. *The Pleasantries of the Incredible Mulla Nasrudin.* New York: E. P. Dutton, 1971.

Simms, Laura. *Stories to Nourish the Hearts of our Children in a Time of Crisis.* New York: n.p., 2001.

---. *Becoming The World.* N.p.: Mercy Corps, 2003.

---. *The Robe of Love: Secret Instructions for the Heart.* New Paltz: Codhill Press, 2002.

Healing Story Alliance – www.healingstory.org

Joseph Campbell Foundation. www.JCF.org

National Storytelling Network – www.storynet.org

Spellbinders Volunteer Storytellers – www.spellbinders.org

Parabola – www.parabola.org

www.aaronshep.com
www.mythinglink.org
www.spiritoftrees.org
www.storycraft.com
www.wisdomtales.com

SUGGESTED READING

Elgin, Duane. *Voluntary Simplicity: Toward a Way of Life that is Outwardly Simple, Inwardly Rich*. New York: William Morrow, 1993.

Estes, Clarissa Pinkola. *Women Who Run With the Wolves: Myths and Stoires of the Wild Woman Archetype*. New York: Ballantine, 1992.

Feinstein, David, and Stanley Krippner. *The Mythic Path: Discovering the Guiding Stories of Your Past — Creating a Vision for your Future*. New York: Jeremy P. Tarcher, Putnam, 1997.

---. *Personal Mythology: Using Ritual, Dreams and Imagination to Discover Your Inner Story*. New York: Jeremy P. Tarcher, Putnam, 1988.

Fox, John. *Poetic Medicine: The Healing Art of Poem-Making*. New York: Jeremy P. Tarcher, Putnam, 1997.

Hollis, James. *Creating a Life: Finding Your Individual Path*. Station Q, Toronto: Inner City Books, 2001.

Johnson, Robert A. *Inner Work: Using Dreams and Active Imagination for Personal Growth*. San Francisco: Harper, 1988.

Keen, Sam, and Anne Valley Fox. *Your Mythic Journey: Finding Meaning in Your Life Through Writing and Storytelling*. New York: Jeremy P. Tarcher, Putnam, 1973.

Muller, Wayne. *Sabbath: Finding Rest, Renewal and Delight in our Busy Lives*. New York: Bantam, 1999.

Weintraub, Amy. *Yoga for Depression: A Compassionate Guide to Relieving Suffering Through Yoga*. New York: Broadway Books, 2004.

STORYTIME YOGA STORY SOURCES

Most of these stories I heard when I was a child and are very common. The following are several sources.

THE RABBIT IN THE MOON – India

Bauer, Caroline Feller. *New Handbook for Storytellers: With stories, poems, magic, and more.* Chicago: ALA, 1993.

White, Rosalyn. *The Rabbit in the Moon.* N.p.: Dharma, 1989.

Adler, Naomi. *Dial book of animal tales from around the world.* New York: Dial Books for Young Readers, 1996.

THE PEDDLER'S DREAM – England

This story has its origins in the 1001 Nights.

The Book of the Thousand Nights and a Night. Trans. Richard F. Burton. London, 1885.

Hartland, Edwin Sidney. *English Fairy and Other Folk Tales.* London, [c. 1890]. 76–77. Hartland's source is the diary of Abraham de la Pryme, Nov. 10, 1699.

Lupton, Hugh. *Tales of Wisdom and Wonder.* Bristol, England: Barefoot Books, 1998.

Another variation:
Diane Wolkstein's *The Magic Orange Tree, and other Haitian folktales.* New York: Knopf, 1978.

A fine version:
Cohelo, Paolo. *The Alchemist.* San Francisco: Harper, 1995.

THE LION'S WHISKER – England

Forrest, Heather. *Wisdom Tales From Around the World.* Little Rock: August House, 1996.

Abdallah, Ali Lutfi. *The Clever Shiek of the Butana and other Stories: Sudanese Folk Tales.* New York: Interlink Books, 1999.

MacDonald, Margaret Read. *Peace Tales: World Folktales to Talk About.* North Haven: Linnet, 1992.

THE MAGIC PEAR TREE – China

Livo, Norma. *Moon Cakes to Maize: Delicious World Folktales*. Golden: Fulcrum, 1999.
Ma, Y.W., and Joseph S.M. Lau, eds. *Traditional Chinese Stories*. New York: Columbia UP, 1978.
Roberts, Moss. *Chinese Fairy Tales and Fantasies*. New York: Pantheon Books, 1979.
Chang, Margaret, and Raymond Chang. *The Beggar's Magic*. New York: Margaret K. McElderry Books, 1997.

DIAMONDS, RUBIES and PEARLS – Germany

I heard this a lot growing up. Children tell me there is a full–length book out there and the story continues. I also heard it from Clarissa Pinkola Estes, Ph.D. It is a variation of the Grimm's Fairy Tale, Mother Hulda.

GANESHA'S LESSON – India

Parabola Magazine. Volume 24, No. 1, 1999.
Krishnaswami, Uma. *The Broken Tusk: Stories of the Hindu God Ganesha*. North Haven: Linnet, 1996.

THE BUFFALO DANCE – Native America

Ewers, John. *The Blackfeet*. Norman: U of Oklahoma P, 1958.
Moyers, Bill, and Joseph Campbell. *The Power of Myth*. New York: Anchor, 1991.
Van Laan, Nancy. *The Buffalo Dance*. Boston: Little, 1993.

Joseph Campbell and the Power of Myth. With Bill Moyers. Mystic Fire Video, 2001.

THE SHIPWRECKED SAILOR – Egypt

The story is found in an ancient papyrus scroll in the Hermitage Museum in Moscow.

Eva March Tappan, ed. *The World's Story: A History of the World in Story, Song and Art*. Boston: Houghton Mifflin, 1914.
Bower, Tamara. *The Shipwrecked Sailor*. New York: Atheneum Books for Young Readers, 2000.
Seton-Williams, M.V. *Egyptian Myths and Legends*. New York: Barnes, 1999.

Namasté

Sydney Solis

Happily

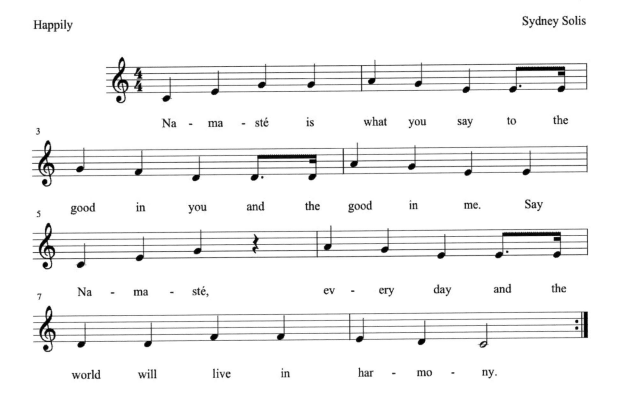

Breathing Song

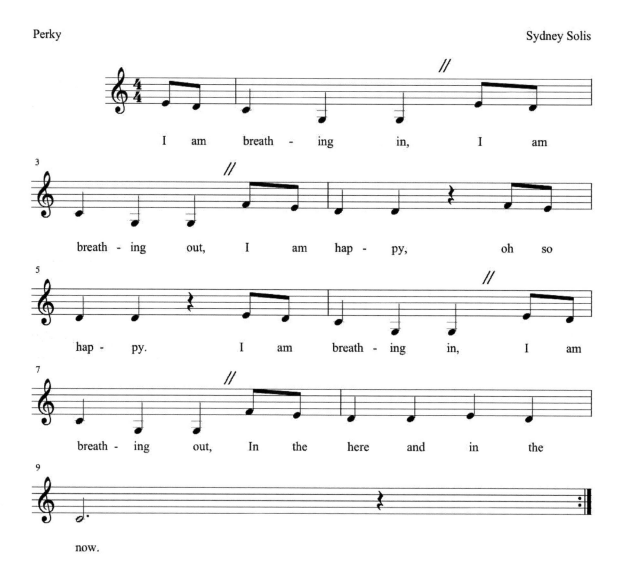

Polar Bear Song

Brightly

Sydney Solis

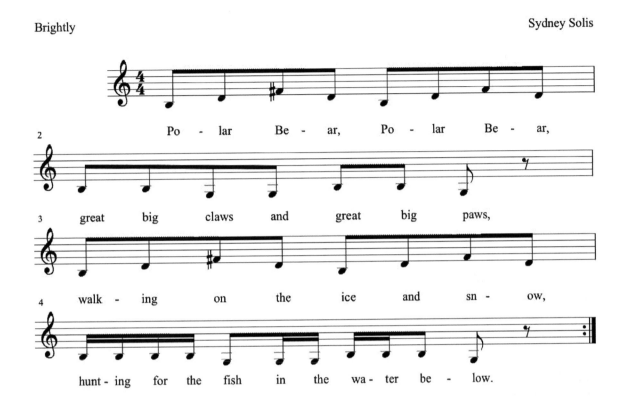

Transcribed by Jennifer Thomas

Cheetah Song

With Energy

Sydney Solis

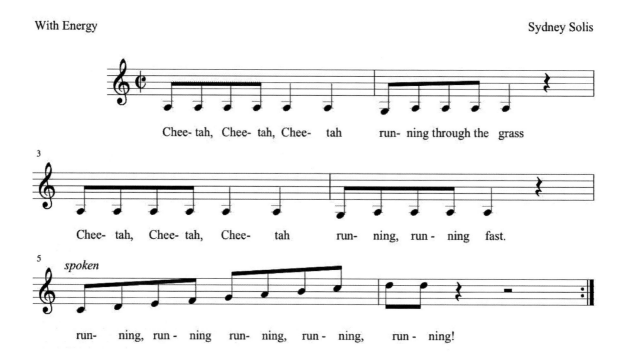

Chee- tah, Chee- tah, Chee- tah   run- ning through the grass

Chee- tah, Chee- tah, Chee-   tah   run- ning, run - ning   fast.

spoken

run- ning, run - ning   run- ning, run - ning,   run - ning!

©Sydney Solis
Transcribed by Jennifer Thomas

I Am Love

Lovingly

Sydney Solis

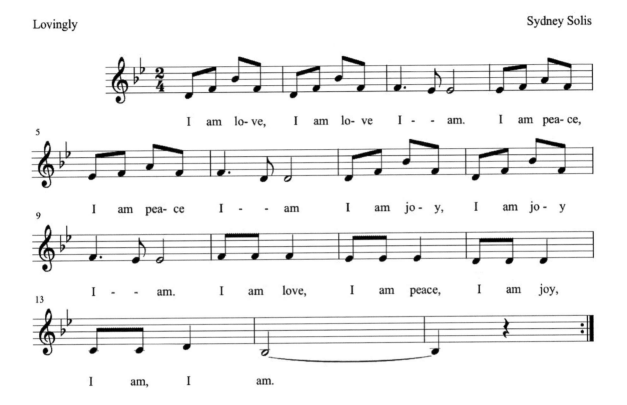

I am lo- ve, I am lo- ve I - - am. I am pea- ce,

I am pea- ce I - - am I am jo- y, I am jo- y

I - - am. I am love, I am peace, I am joy,

I am, I am.

Transcribed by Jennifer Thomas

ABOUT THE AUTHOR

Sydney Solis grew up in Boulder, Colorado, and studied theater and dance at the University of Colorado and did workstudy with the Nancy Spanier Dance Theatre. She received a B.A. in journalism and Spanish from Metropolitan State College of Denver and worked as a journalist and award–winning photographer in Colorado, California, Mexico and Ecuador.

She became a storyteller in 2000, and was a Spellbinder volunteer storyteller in the public schools. Her professional premier was in 2004 at the Rocky Mountain Storytellers' Conference with *The Golden Cucumber, Stories from Indonesia,* which is also a storytelling CD. She is also co–author of *Hot Today, Gone Tamale and other Tummy Tales.*

She has performed at numerous storytelling festivals, libraries, schools and conferences in Colorado and nationally. She teaches storytelling and yoga classes, and workshops for children and adults nationally, including the Healing Through Story Conference and the League for the Advancement of New England Storytelling.

Sydney has worked as an English as a Second Language tutor in public elementary and high schools and spent seven years working in her children's Montessori classrooms. She has also volunteered with the Kern County California Health Department and taught adult literacy.

She is an associate of the Joseph Campbell Foundation and hosts JCF roundtable gatherings throughout Colorado. For more information visit ww.JCF.org.

She is the widowed mother of two small children and lives in a little house with a big garden and two cats in Boulder, Colorado.

For more information, see her web sites at:

www.MythicYoga.com
www.StorytimeYoga.com